your happy baby

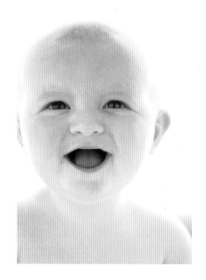

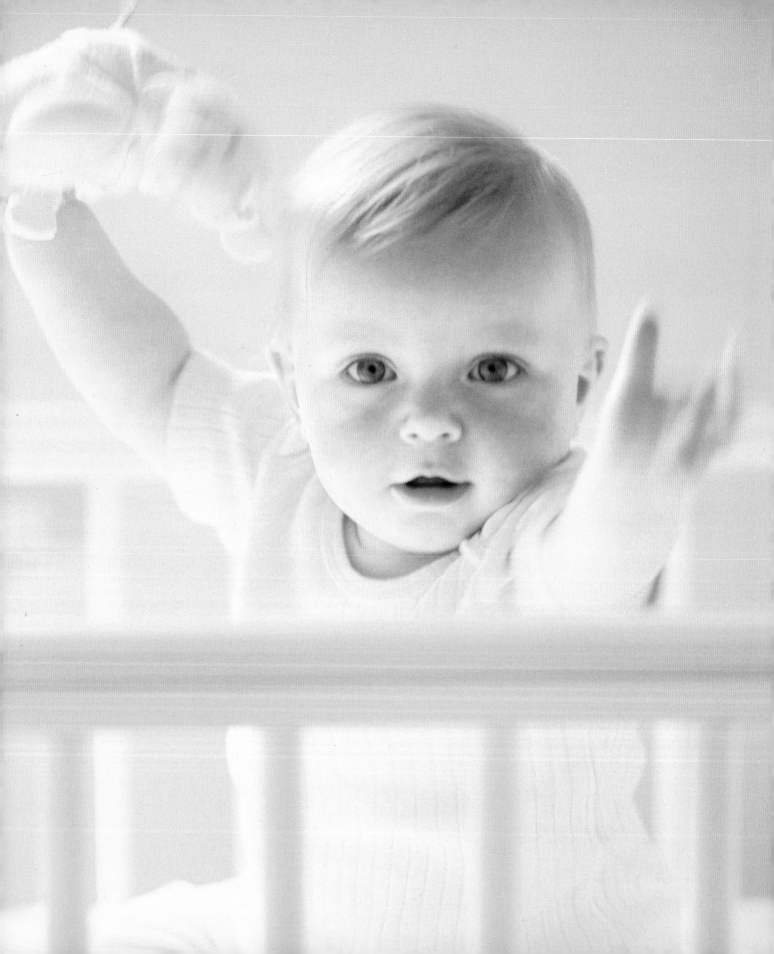

your happy baby

massage, yoga, aromatherapy and
other gentle ways to blissful babyhood

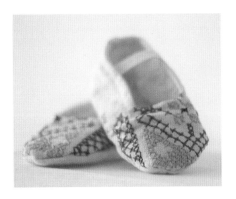

contributing editor
Sheena Meredith

contributing authors
Tina Lam, Clare Mundy *and* Glenda Taylor

with photography by Dan Duchars

RYLAND
PETERS
& SMALL

LONDON NEW YORK

SENIOR DESIGNER Sonya Nathoo

SENIOR EDITOR Henrietta Heald

LOCATION RESEARCH Tracy Ogino

PRODUCTION MANAGER Patricia Harrington

ART DIRECTOR Anne-Marie Bulat

EDITORIAL DIRECTOR Julia Charles

PUBLISHING DIRECTOR Alison Starling

First published in the UK in 2006 by
Ryland Peters & Small
20–21 Jockey's Fields
London WC1R 4BW
www.rylandpeters.com

10 9 8 7 6 5 4 3 2 1

ISBN-10: 1-84597-129-9
ISBN-13: 978-1-84597-129-8

A CIP record for this book is available from
the British Library.

Printed and bound in China.

**Neither the authors nor the publisher can be
held responsible for any claim arising out of the
use or misuse of suggestions made in this book.
While every effort has been made to ensure
that the information contained in the book is
accurate and up to date, it is advisory only and
should not be used as an alternative to seeking
specialist medical advice.**

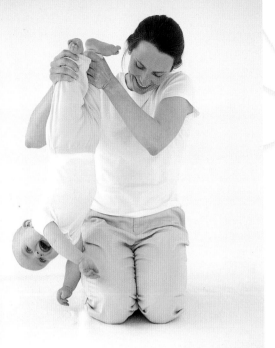

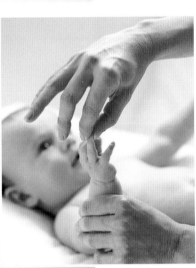

contents

introduction

As any experienced mother will tell you, babies are little for only a very short while – or so you realize afterwards. It probably won't seem so at the time, especially if this is your first baby. You may even feel overwhelmed by your experience of motherhood, wondering how one small person can create such chaos in a household, or require so much care and attention.

By looking at the things that affect a baby's happiness and suggesting myriad ways to understand your baby better, *Your Happy Baby* will help you to make the most of the precious weeks and months of your child's babyhood. Starting with the birth, here are techniques you can use to get to know each other, have fun and create a time that you will always look back on with joy.

Even an uncomplicated birth is a huge event both physically and emotionally. It's natural to need some time to recover. You won't ever 'get back to normal' because 'normal' has changed, but we offer some useful hints for being kind to yourself and to your baby as you move towards an established routine in your new life together. The book also covers some of the special circumstances that you may face, such as a premature or caesarean birth.

Your Happy Baby includes expert advice and practical instruction on physical techniques to promote calm and well-being. You can learn how to avoid or solve feeding problems and how to help your baby – and yourself – to get

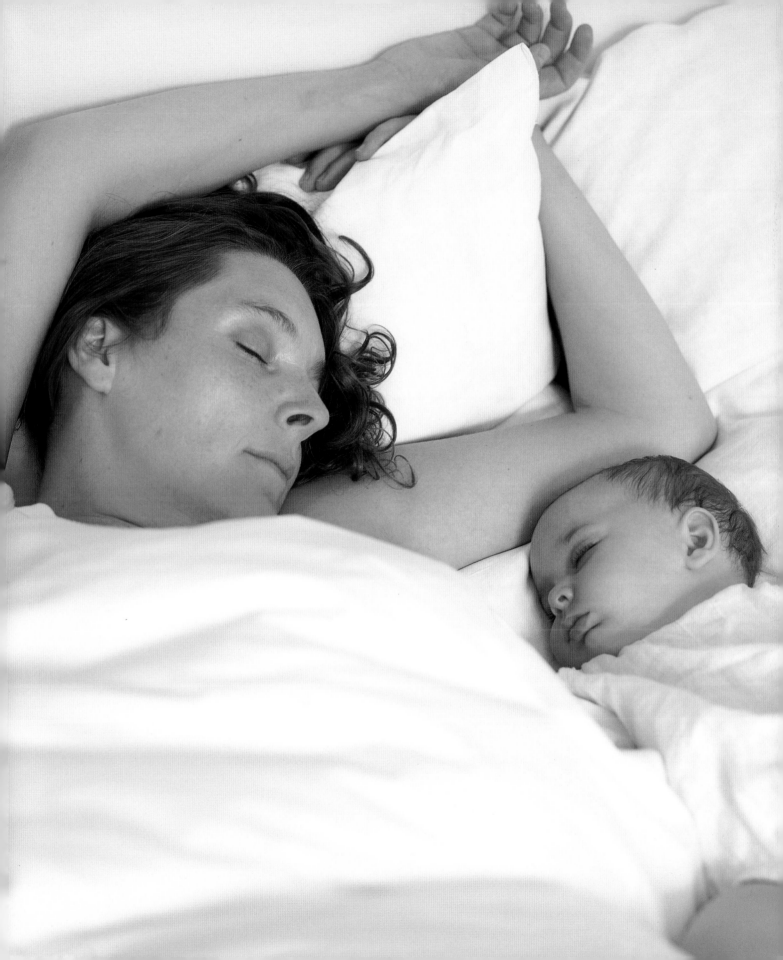

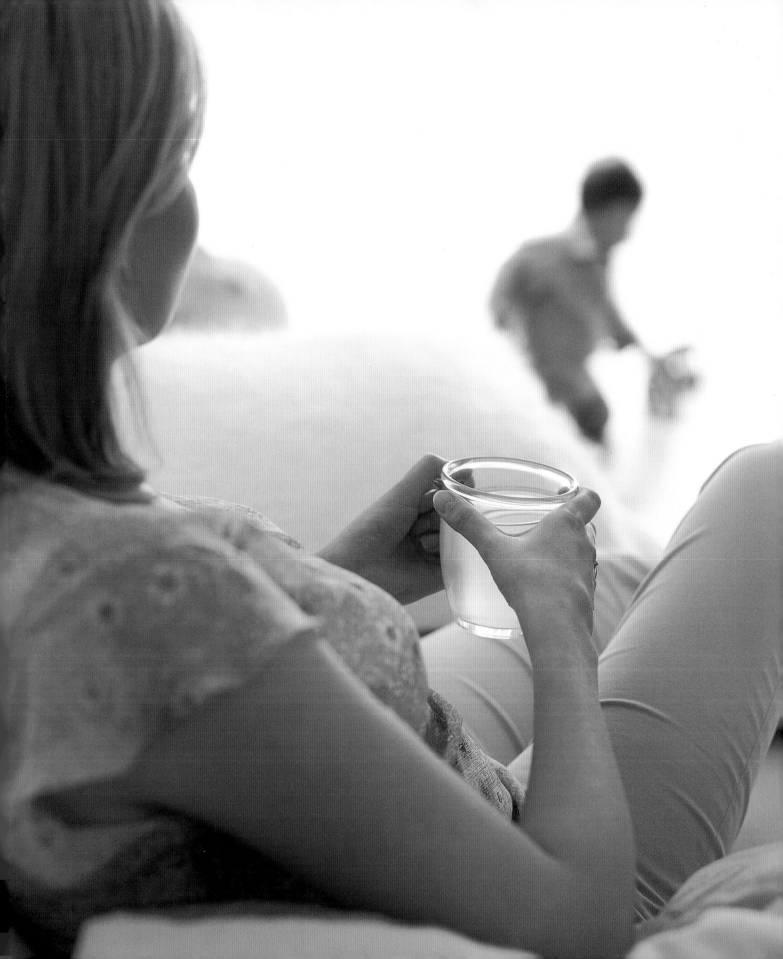

a good night's sleep more quickly. We will show you how to massage your baby, describe enjoyable exercises in baby yoga and gym to develop physical skills and protect posture, and suggest ways of using water and aromatherapy to enhance your baby's experience of his or her environment. As you use these techniques, you are communicating with your baby in vital ways – emotionally and verbally as well as physically – and learning your baby's body language and signals. You will soon be able to interpret signs of distress, to soothe when necessary, and to relish smiles and chuckles together.

As well as explaining the gentle therapies of cranial osteopathy, reflexology, homeopathy and Bach Flower Remedies, *Your Happy Baby* also includes advice on natural remedies that can help to soothe or treat minor ailments and prevent some problems from occurring in the first place. Some therapies you can try at home; for others, you will need to seek professional advice.

This book shows how to give your child the best start in life. It will allow you to satisfy your baby's needs, soothe hurt feelings and deal with minor health problems. Just as important, you will have fun creating a loving and stimulating environment. Not only will you enjoy the precious time of babyhood, but also you will start to build your relationship in positive ways that will last for years to come. For you, this relationship will be lifelong. For both of you, it is one of the most important you will ever have. Take time to enjoy it.

SHEENA MEREDITH

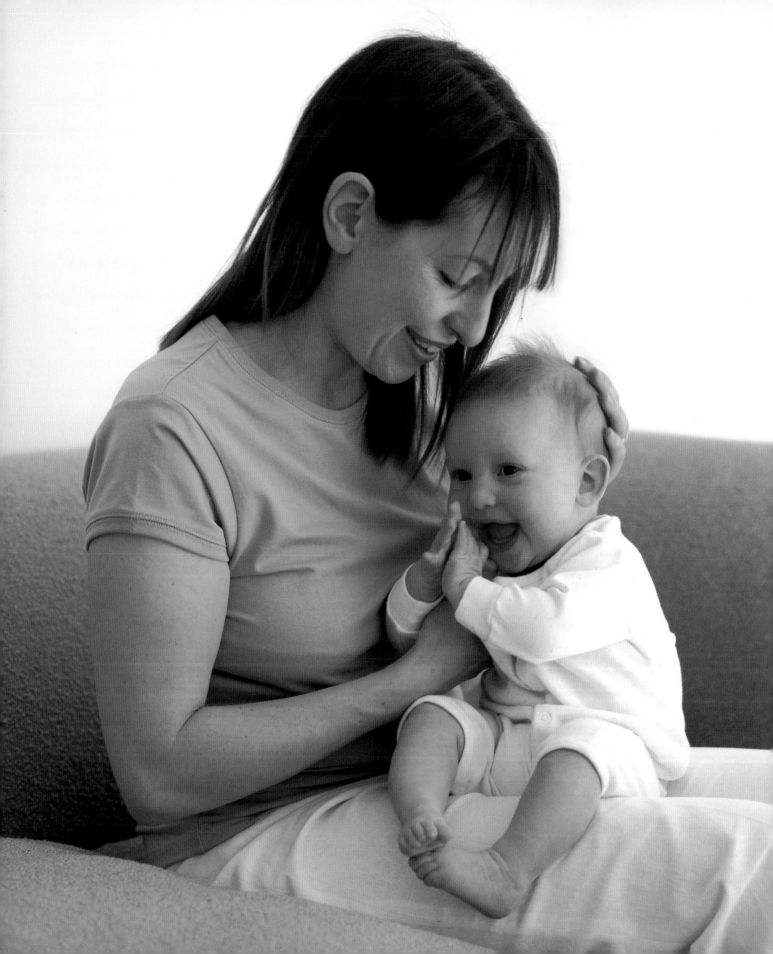

the keys to happiness

Since babies are completely dependent, their physical needs are closely linked with emotional needs for love, comfort and security. So every task of parenthood becomes a labour of love, and every interaction is an opportunity to promote happiness – from an intimate feeding experience to a nappy change with a tickle and a chuckle.

what makes a baby happy?

One of the first things that concerns new parents, apart from the safety and health of their baby, is how to interpret what their baby wants. Babies' communication is limited – which is why crying is geared to be a big attention-grabber – but their sensitivity and capacity to react to their surroundings are boundless.

LOVE AND SECURITY

Assuming that babies have no physical problems, the greatest influence on their happiness is their parents and the other people close to them. A contented mother or father is the best gift that a newborn baby can receive: you will transmit feelings of love, security and confidence, and be more alert, attuned and able to respond to your baby's needs, making parenthood a more joyful experience. So always remember to love, value and nurture yourself as well as your baby.

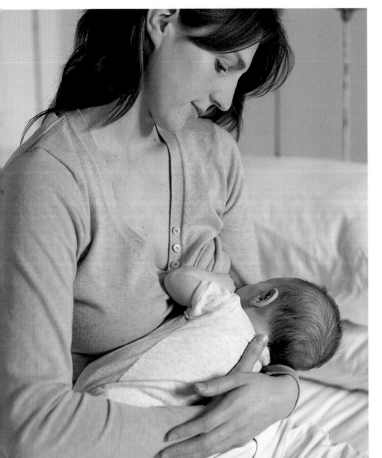

EARLY EXPERIENCES

We are only just beginning to appreciate how much early life events – and events that occur in the womb before birth – can affect our babies' development, emotionally and psychologically as well as physically. Women's concerns about the growth in 'high-tech' hospital births, with high rates of medical intervention, are increasingly reflected in suggestions that modern birthing methods can be stressful for babies, too, with potentially long-lasting effects.

Many women are now seeking gentler births with less intervention. Following on from this has been a growing interest in kinder approaches to childrearing, and a resurgence of traditional practices that involve close physical contact such as baby massage, swaddling, prolonged breastfeeding and co-sleeping.

This book describes gentle activities and therapies that can boost your baby's happiness and explains how to foster a strong emotional bond with your baby from the early days, even if the experience of birth has been less than ideal. It begins by looking at communication.

INTERPRETING YOUR BABY'S NEEDS

One of your top priorities in the early weeks of your baby's life will be learning to decipher the baby's cries. If your baby is wailing and you are not sure why, consider that he or she may be:

☐ Hungry.

☐ Lonely or bored and wanting a cuddle.

☐ In need of a nappy change.

'What became clearer to me after the birth of each of my children was that babies don't need splendid nursery decorations or expensive toys — the only thing that really counts is your love and attention.'

JOANNA, MOTHER OF YASMIN, LOUISE AND ALISTAIR

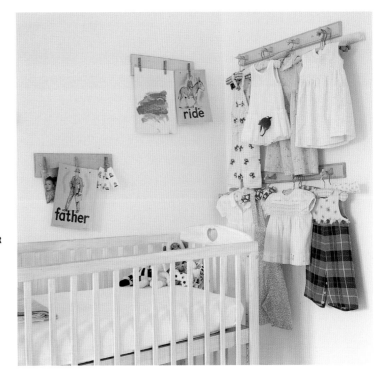

□ Tired. Try to recognize the signs of tiredness before your baby gets overtired – for example, rubbing the eyes, pulling at the ears or a 'grizzly' cry.

□ Too hot, too cold, suffering from wind, or reacting to uncomfortable clothing.

□ Frustrated – especially when meeting new challenges such as trying to roll over, crawl or sit up.

□ Unwell (see pages 114–22).

□ Overstimulated. Some babies can't tolerate excessive noise and activity (others thrive on them).

□ Stressed. Your baby may react against loud noises, nasty smells, family arguments or a parent feeling upset or harassed.

WHAT YOU CAN DO

If you can't work out what's wrong, try carrying your baby close to your chest, rocking or swinging gently as you move around. Try gentle patting or rubbing; some babies like to be tickled. Sing, play music or indulge in touching games such as 'This Little Piggy' and 'Round and Round the Garden'. Sucking can be calming – offer a clean finger, a dummy or a teething toy. Some babies find it soothing to be swaddled – tightly wrapped to restrict arm and leg movements, which may mimic conditions in the womb. Or your baby may be soothed by background noise such as the sound of a working washing machine or vacuum cleaner, or movement such as that generated by going for a drive in a car.

A screaming baby can make more noise than a road drill – and continual exposure to such noise can lead to parental stress and depression. Give yourself a break. If you have done all you can, put the baby in a safe place and leave the room. Sit quietly, sip a hot drink, breathe fresh air, meditate – whatever it takes to clear the mind and calm the spirit. If you achieve this, you will have more to offer your baby when you return to the fray.

NOURISHMENT

Your feeding choices will affect your child's health from birth through to adulthood. Breastfeeding protects against infections, allergies, obesity and many diseases. (It also protects you against breast cancer and helps you to lose weight gained in pregnancy). Breast milk is instantly available, portable, warm, sterile – and free. And breastfeeding brings you and your baby closer. So breastfeed if you possibly can.

It helps to have support from the start – ideally, your baby should be put to the breast within an hour of the birth. Check your midwife's attitude to breastfeeding in advance, if you can. If you have problems with feeding, get help fast before giving up; most difficulties can be resolved. Your local La Leche League counsellor (see page 124) will give advice at any time.

However, if for any reason you cannot breastfeed, don't feel bad about it – your baby will sense it. There are many other good things about your relationship, so focus on making bottle-feeding as close and magical an experience as you can – hold your baby lovingly and take this time together to gaze into each other's eyes.

Although any breastfeeding is better than none, your baby will benefit most if you breastfeed exclusively for six months. If possible, feed on demand – whenever your baby wants to. Offer your breast at the first hint of hunger, such as squirming or chewing fingers; crying is a late sign. All babies have their own rhythms and may sometimes simply need the comfort of sucking. Unless you live in the tropics, your baby needs nothing else, not even water. Solid foods can be given from around the age of six months. Ideally, try to continue breastfeeding as well until your baby is at least a year old – if you do not, your baby will need formula milk as a substitute. The longer breastfeeding continues, the greater the benefits. In any event, take weaning slowly or your baby and your breasts will protest.

Many babies wean themselves, gradually dropping feeds when they are ready; the bedtime feed is usually the last to go. If given the opportunity, children may breastfeed well into toddlerhood.

When you introduce solids, remember that eating habits developed now will last a lifetime. Set a good example and provide healthy meals for the whole family (that way, your baby can eat the same foods, chopped or liquidized). If you offer something that your baby doesn't like, wait a few weeks and introduce it again in a different form – for example, stewed rather than puréed apple or apple with blackcurrants. Bright colours, such as small pieces of chopped fruit and vegetables, can often tempt fussy eaters.

SUCCESSFUL BREASTFEEDING

Breastfeeding is much more likely to succeed if you are relaxed and your baby is in the right position to latch onto the nipple easily. Make yourself comfortable – whenever possible, pick a pleasant, calm environment and a comfortable chair. Have everything you may need within easy reach: a drink, reading material, an object for meditation, the telephone if necessary.

Always bring your baby's mouth up to nipple height – if you lean over, you may end up with sore nipples,

don't forget to **look at your baby** during feeds — feeding

offers a wonderful opportunity to **get close** to

your baby and to **strengthen the bond** between you

backache and shoulder strain. Use pillows or cushions to raise your baby on your lap, so that the baby is lying sideways facing your breast with the head cradled in the crook of your arm. Make sure your elbows and back are well supported, and prop your feet on a foot rest. To begin with, it may be easier to settle yourself first and have someone pass your baby to you.

Support your breast so that it is not pressing on your baby's chin and gently guide the nipple and areola into your baby's mouth – it should be wide open, to take in at least half an inch of the areola (the dark area surrounding the nipple). If you feel any discomfort or pain, gently insert a clean little finger between your baby's gums and your nipple, and start again. When the position is right, it should feel quite comfortable, and you will soon see sucking movements of the jaw. It is crucial that your baby latches onto the nipple properly – if you are in any doubt, seek advice early.

Once you are accustomed to breastfeeding, you will be able to vary the positions in which you feed.

COMFORT, SAFETY AND STIMULATION

There are many things you can do to affect your baby's surroundings and early experiences in order to increase his sense of security and contentment. A calm, pleasant environment is much more important than lots of toys.

□ Babies like warmth; dress them in one more layer of clothing than you are wearing, but make sure that they do not become too hot.

□ Since babies put everything in their mouths, toys and playthings should all be clean and washable.

□ Examine all toys for choking, strangling or trapping hazards before giving them to your baby.

□ Safety first! Look at your home from your baby's level before he or she begins to crawl.

□ Involve your baby in family life from the start.

□ Talk to your baby as much as possible. Explain what you are doing, name things, point to parts of the body.

Mothers naturally use a special tone of voice – 'baby talk' – but avoid baby words such as choo-choo and bow-wow, or your baby will have to learn names twice.

□ Encourage your baby to appreciate nature – point out trees, birds, clouds.

□ Stimulate all the senses – give your baby different things to look at, hear, touch, taste and smell.

□ Sing or play music. Babies like rhythm and repetition – lullabies, nursery rhymes, clapping games.

□ Encourage exercise from an early age.

PARENTAL CONFIDENCE

Above all, have confidence in your abilities as a parent. Modern parents receive perhaps too much advice from professionals, yet are often given too little support. So trust your instincts, take help when it's offered, and ask for more if you feel overwhelmed. Most importantly, remember that your child's babyhood will soon be gone – enjoy it together.

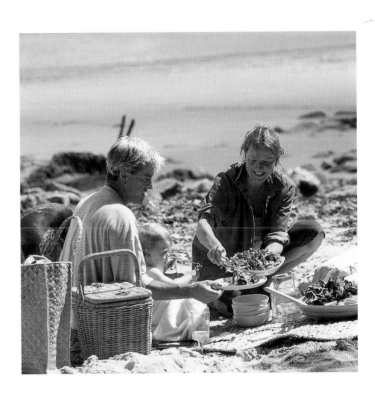

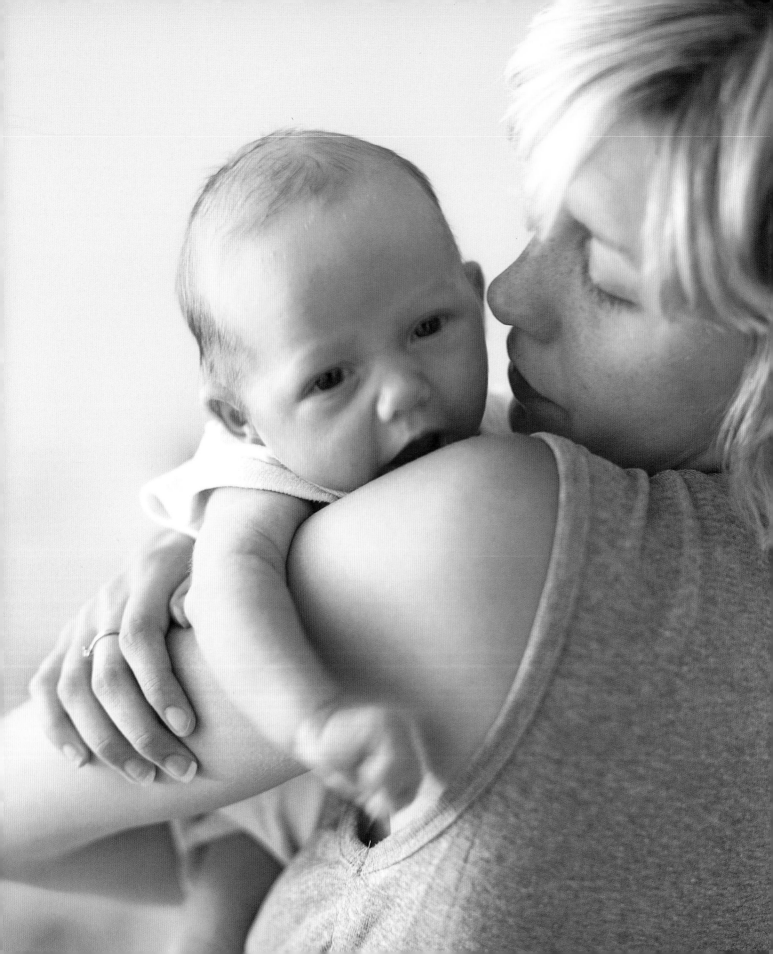

coming into the world

There will never be a greater transition. In the womb, your baby was held securely, bathed in warm fluid, rocked by your movements and soothed by your heartbeats. Then the momentous journey of labour begins . . .

A RUDE AWAKENING

As contractions progress and labour builds up towards its climax, the baby is being squeezed with increasing pressure, twisted in the birth canal and pushed out of a familiar cosy environment. Suddenly the baby arrives in the air, and has to breathe with lungs for the first time. Light floods the baby's eyes, and unusual noises and unfamiliar smells bombard the senses. Soon the baby will meet other challenges in adapting to a whole new world. Who knows what he or she feels – whether or not the experience is frightening, it is certainly stressful.

To make your baby's arrival as calm as possible, try to retain as much control as you can over the moment of birth. Minimize the shock to your baby by keeping lights dimmed and the sound level low. Delay cutting the cord. Hold your baby as soon as possible. If you had a drug-free birth, make the most of the alert period in the hour or so after birth. For other ways to help your baby to make a good start in life, see pages 20–21.

LOVING TOUCH AND 'KANGAROO CARE'

The trauma of birth and its aftermath is felt even more keenly by premature babies, who often spend the first days or weeks of life in a neonatal intensive care unit, deprived of the comforting sensations of touch, while being subjected to handling that may be experienced as intrusive and disturbing. In addition, much of what goes on happens irrespective of any signals the baby makes. A premature baby lacks control over his or her environment even more than a full-term baby. Yet soothing physical contact and loving touch in the early days of life are vital for later growth and development.

In many countries where intensive care is unavailable, premature infants are given 'kangaroo care'. They are carried upright and naked, apart from a nappy, against the parent's bare chest, with their head turned to hear mother's or father's heartbeat. Prolonged skin-to-skin contact helps to regulate temperature, breathing and heartbeat, improves weight gain, reduces hospital stay, and more than doubles survival rates. Even in full-term infants, such carrying lessens crying, improves sleeping, promotes breastfeeding and may reduce colic.

So touch, stroke and cuddle your baby as much as possible, and try to respond to any cues. If your baby enjoys hearing a lullaby, for example, keep singing.

OVERSTIMULATION

Another way in which premature babies give an insight into early life is in their reaction to external stimuli. A relatively disorganized nervous system means that they are easily overstimulated by noises or sights. Signs of this include turning the face away, crying or squirming.

If you have a newborn who behaves in this way, tone down visual stimuli, reduce the noise level, dim lights and give the baby time to cope. Think carefully about what's around your baby: garish, brightly coloured or noisy items may be especially unsuitable. Choose soft pastel colours, gentle sounds and slow-moving objects. Once your infant is a little older and more robust, baby massage may be helpful (see pages 22–51).

caesarean births

Whether a caesarean section was planned or happened after difficulties in labour, caesarean babies face special problems adapting. It can be hard to support your baby through this period when you yourself are recovering from a major operation. Be aware that both of you will need extra time and masses of love and support.

PHYSICAL EFFECTS

Caesarean babies often have more rounded heads than babies born vaginally, who can appear rather squashed, but they may have problems simply because the birth was sudden and the head did not undergo the normal moulding process during its journey through the birth canal. Cranial osteopaths believe that this can result in various imbalances (see pages 104–105), and you may wish to see a practitioner to correct these.

Caesarean babies are often premature, are more vulnerable to respiratory distress and may be affected by what prompted the operation. Occasionally, they may have been cut accidentally, or, rarely, a joint may be dislocated. A baby with physical problems needs extra attention, and you may need help to cope with sleeping or feeding problems.

DRUGS

After a general anaesthetic, you and your baby will be drowsy and lethargic for a while. There is less risk from an epidural, but some of the drug is absorbed into the bloodstream, where it may interfere with oxytocin (a hormone important in breastfeeding and bonding), and some reaches the baby through the placenta. Little is known about the effects on babies, although breathing difficulties and low blood sugar have been reported.

Often the mother will be given painkillers and antibiotics after a caesarean, and a breastfed baby will be exposed to tiny amounts of these drugs as well.

A baby's immature system can have trouble expelling these drugs, so effects may last several days. Antibiotics can also cause yeast infections – vaginal thrush in the mother and sometimes thrush in the baby's mouth or groin; the mother's nipples may be affected during feeding. Watch for redness, soreness and white patches – and seek rapid treatment if they develop.

RECOVERY

A big drawback of caesarean section is separation from your baby immediately after birth. A hospital stay of at least four to five days also delays your ability to care for your baby without help and separates both of you from the rest of your family. Once back at home, you will find it painful to move around for a while, making caring for a new baby harder. It can take longer to bond with your baby, but be patient – it will happen.

BREASTFEEDING

Your milk may take longer to come in after a caesarean and the baby may find it hard to latch on, especially if there are sore patches from the suction tube usually put in a baby's mouth after birth. You may also find it more difficult to get into a comfortable position. Try holding the baby under one arm like a rugby ball, with a rolled towel placed over the wound to avoid pain. Breastfeeding generally takes longer to establish after a caesarean – but is well worth the effort for both of you. If necessary, seek professional advice (see page 124).

soothing physical contact and **loving touch** in the early days of life are vital for later **healthy growth** and **emotional and psychological** development

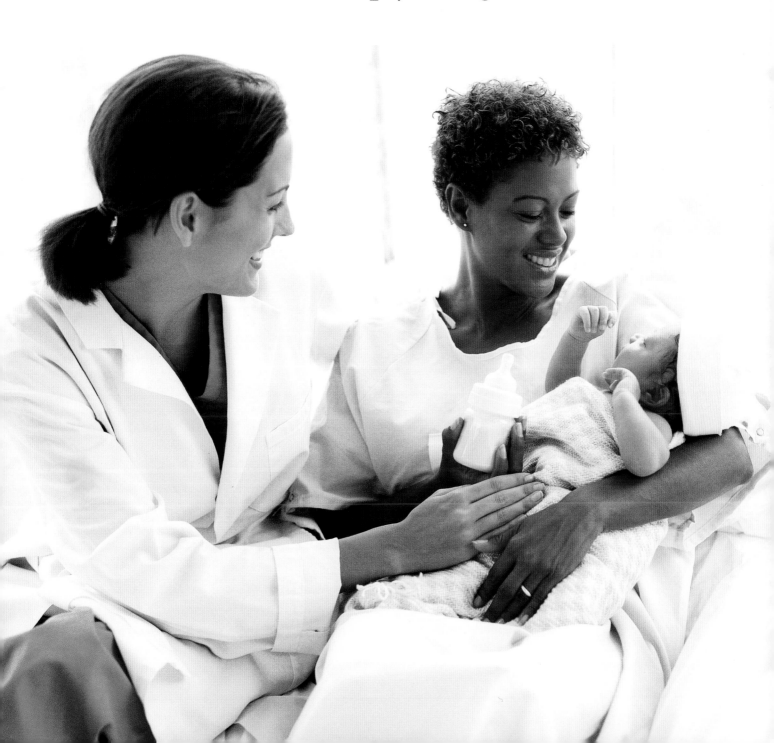

Although none of us can remember it, the experience of being born is one of the most challenging physical and psychological ordeals that we must undergo. There are many things that you can do to minimize the shock of birth and to give your baby a happy start in life.

TEN WAYS TO... *make a good start*

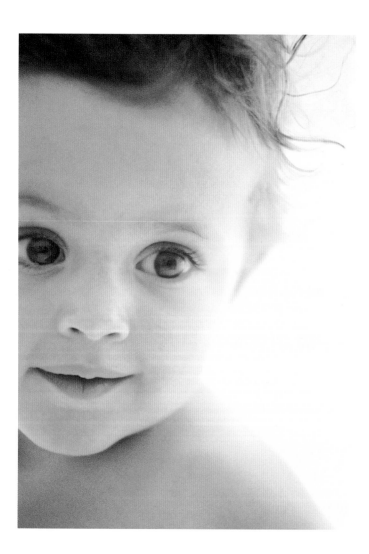

I Establish an atmosphere of calm in the birthing room by asking for the lights to be kept dimmed and the sound level kept low; if possible, have a soothing, familiar piece of music playing in the background.

2 Don't bathe your baby too soon after the birth. Babies are born with a thin covering of a white, greasy substance called vernix to protect their skin in the womb (imagine being in a warm bath for nine months!). After birth, the vernix protects against infection and helps to maintain body temperature. A few days later it is absorbed into the skin.

3 Breastfeed your baby as soon as possible. Ideally, put your baby to your breast immediately after birth – as well as being soothing, this will give you a hormone boost that encourages the womb to keep contracting and helps the expulsion of the placenta (the third stage of labour). Feeding on demand – that is, whenever your baby wants to – ensures that your baby never goes hungry and always has a source of comfort. Your breasts will produce as much milk as your baby needs. If for any reason you are unable to breastfeed, make bottle-feeding as close and loving an experience as you can.

4 Hold your baby close to your chest as much as possible. Skin-to-skin contact is the ultimate comfort, and baby massage encourages closeness.

5 Respond to your baby's cries. Crying is a newborn's only method of communication and you will neither spoil the baby nor encourage crying by reacting to it. Indeed, research has shown that babies whose needs are met more quickly seem to cry less.

6 Don't use bath or skin-care products for the first month or two – they're not necessary and may clog your baby's delicate skin and disrupt the development of protective skin acids (babies are born with alkaline skin). This can encourage spots, cradle cap, nappy rash, infections and allergies. Meanwhile plain water and cotton wool for washing is fine.

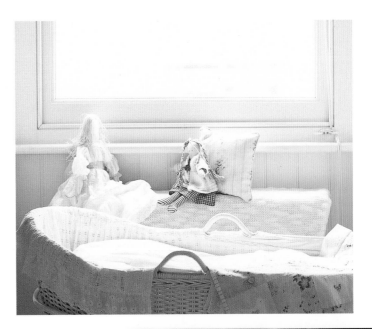

7 Stare at your baby – you may find that you do this by instinct. Although babies' vision is blurry, they can see anything up to two feet away, and what they want to see most is your face. Your baby will probably gaze adoringly back.

8 Keep your baby's environment quiet and soothing for the first few weeks. Avoid too many visitors (unless they have come to help) – this will also protect your baby against infections.

9 Consider swaddling your baby. Tight wrapping is a traditional form of comfort for babies – the feeling of being cocooned may mimic the conditions of the womb and make the baby feel safe.

10 If your baby has any physical problems resulting from the birth, consider consulting a cranial osteopath or a homeopath for treatment or advice (see pages 104–105 and 108–109).

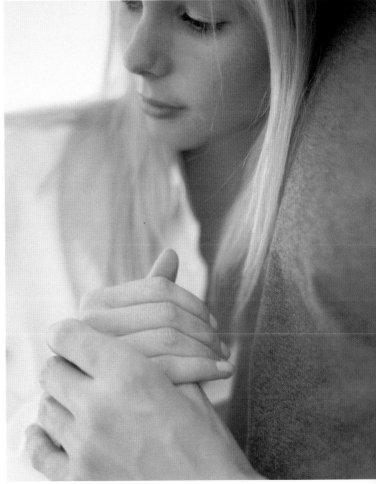

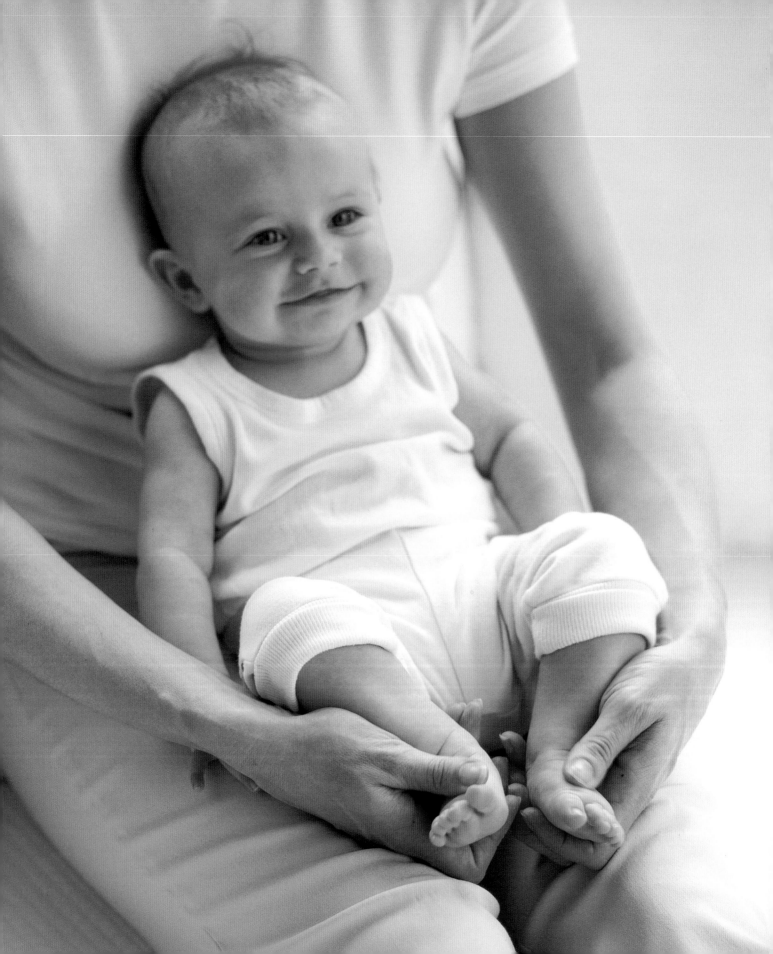

baby massage

Massage is one of the most delightful and effective physical therapies you can share with your baby, and one of the easiest to learn. So switch off the phone and, with the simplest of preparations, treat your baby and yourself to this loving touch that will leave you both feeling peaceful, happy and thoroughly refreshed.

massage: the principles

If you are new to baby massage, you will be learning step by step, and so will your baby: a few basic principles will get you started on the right track, and after that it's a matter of intuition – and practice.

RECOVERING FROM BIRTH

Stroking and soothing babies by rubbing them with oil is an age-old practice that, in various parts of the world, has been passed down through generations without even being given a name. Often the midwife or woman in attendance will massage not only the newborn child but also the baby's mother for up to ten days after the birth, helping both of them to recover from labour.

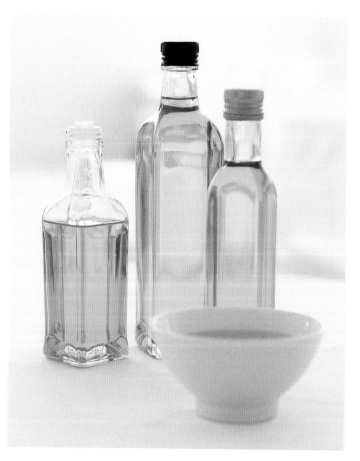

THE BENEFITS FOR BABIES. . .

Regular massage helps babies to recover from birth by reducing stress levels and boosting feel-good hormones such as oxytocin, the bonding hormone also produced by nursing mothers. Massage has also been shown to help babies born pre-term to gain weight. As well as encouraging good sleeping patterns, it can be used to relieve wind, colic, constipation and pain from teething.

. . . AND FOR THEIR PARENTS

Nor are the benefits of massage reserved for babies alone. Mothers who massage their babies experience swifter recovery from any postnatal depression, a reduction in blood pressure and heart rate, and the release of serotonin, a 'natural opiate' that makes us feel relaxed and cheerful. Fathers, too, find that gentle hands-on contact with their babies is an important way to feel involved in parenting right from the start.

TIME TO ENJOY

First and foremost, however, baby massage is about taking the time to enjoy some precious moments each day with your baby. Loving touch is a form of intuition – literally, teaching from within – through which we learn again what we already know but have forgotten.

It is a very special process, during which you find out what your baby likes, and even who she is, through observation and spending time together. Quieten your mind, let go of tension in your body, and experience the well-being that flows from what has been described as 'the ultimate cuddle' with your baby.

'Paolo was born prematurely and he only started gaining weight properly when I began to give him regular massage.'

ANA, MOTHER OF PAOLO

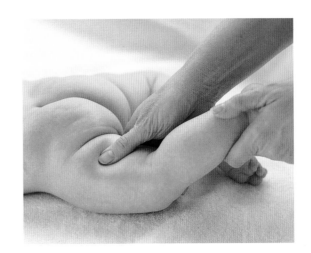

WHAT YOU NEED

Your baby will probably be unclothed for the massage, so the first essential is a warm room. The recommended temperature for baby massage is 26°C (80°F), although babies with eczema respond better to a slightly cooler environment. Make sure your hands are warm, too.

Maintaining eye contact with your baby as you massage will reassure him that you are responsive to his needs. Babies tend to be fascinated by light and will stare at windows – so keep the room shaded from too much bright light to help you to focus on each other.

WHICH OILS?

The type of oil you choose for massage is up to you. Babies sometimes taste the oil by putting their hands to their mouth, so a natural edible oil such as sunflower or grapeseed is a good solution; these oils are light and will be absorbed into your baby's skin during massage, helping to moisturize any dry spots. Other good oils include what is known as fractionated coconut oil (which is light and liquid) and other vegetable-based oils, especially avocado.

You will require about 50ml oil for each massage, poured into a shallow bowl. A 500ml bottle of oil should be enough for ten massages. For the sake of good hygiene, dispose of the used oil afterwards. For more information on suitable oils, see the chapter on Baby Aromatherapy (pages 84–99).

Some baby massage oils and gels contain other ingredients such as perfume that may affect your baby's delicate skin, so test for an allergic reaction before embarking on a full massage. The first time you use any type of oil on your baby's skin, massage only the feet for five to ten minutes. The usual allergic reaction is a sudden blotchiness or an obvious reddening of the skin; if you notice something similar on your baby's feet, simply wash off the oil with plenty of soap and water.

HOW MUCH PRESSURE?

Babies respond well to a degree of pressure when being massaged. As a rough guide, use the same amount of pressure as you would when shampooing your hair, but in the first few weeks of your baby's life keep pressure very light – no heavier than the pressure you would apply to your eyeballs with the lids closed.

Providing you apply plenty of oil when you massage a baby (to reduce friction), you can press and squeeze soft tissue and muscle – but stroke more gently over bony areas. Too light a touch will tickle your baby and make him tense up – the opposite effect to relaxing!

positions and equipment

Therapeutic massage practitioners work at a table that is the correct height to protect their back from strain. It is important to get into a comfortable position before you massage your baby – one in which your shoulders, arms and hands are fully relaxed and your lower back is supported.

GETTING COMFORTABLE

The safest place to massage your baby is when sitting on the floor. On a wooden floor you will need a non-slip mat to sit on. Wear something loose and stretchy that allows you to lean forward and move about freely. An alternative to sitting is to stand at a table which is high enough so that you do not have to lean over too much.

There are three positions suggested here – try each in turn to see which works best for you. Baby massage should be relaxing for you both – if you feel awkward or uncomfortable, you will have tension in your upper body, shoulders and hands and this will communicate itself to your baby. Don't be afraid to stop massaging for a moment to alter your position, if you need to.

POSITION ONE

Sit as shown below, with your legs together and your lower back up against a firm supporting surface such

'The sitting position was useful to learn since – unlike kneeling and leaning forward – it is perfectly comfortable.'

MARIE, MOTHER OF ERIN

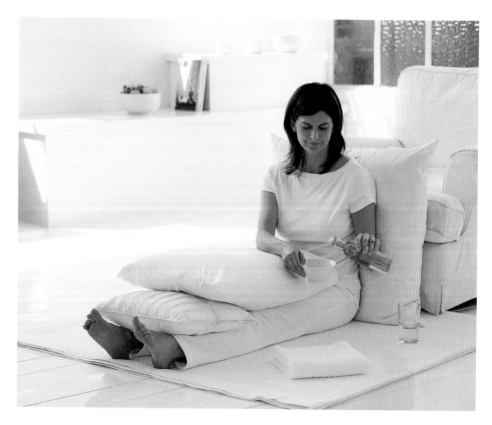

as a wall or furniture that will not move. Push yourself back so that you are resting upright on your 'sitting bones' rather than slouching. This will enable you to lean forward without strain. Place the pillow on your legs, with a small cushion on your ankles so that the pillow does not slope away from you.

POSITION TWO

You will find this comfortable if you have flexibility in your hips and pelvis. Sit against a support with your legs apart and the pillow on the floor between them. (There is no need for a cushion because the pillow will be level.) Bend your knees a little if you like, letting them fall outwards so they do not prevent you from leaning forward. Again, protect your back from strain by keeping it straight and leaning forward from the hips.

POSITION THREE

People with flexible knee joints may find it comfortable to sit cross-legged. As in the other two positions, make sure that you have adequate support for your lower back. You will need two pillows, one resting on top of the other; bring the top one closer to you, as shown below. Place the small cushion under the top pillow if necessary to keep it level.

WHAT YOU WILL NEED

The basic equipment for baby massage is as follows:

□ A large towel.
□ One or two pillows.
□ One small cushion and one medium-sized cushion.
□ Massage oil.
□ A ceramic or glass bowl.
□ Tissues.

The towel should be long enough to cover the pillow, with some spare folds in your lap for mopping up spills and leaks. Massage will relax all your baby's internal organs, including the bladder! The medium-sized cushion is useful for an older baby who wants to sit up (see Becoming Mobile, pages 48–49).

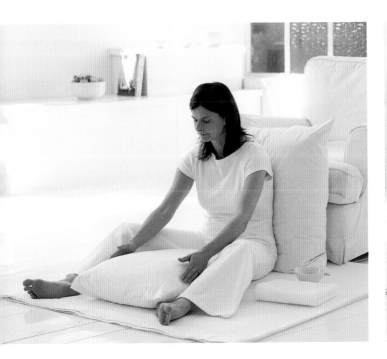

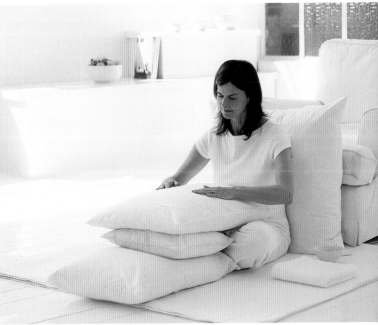

massage techniques

Although the massage strokes described on these pages are called techniques, there is nothing mysterious about them – and you will probably, perhaps unconsciously, have done most of them already.

DISCOVERING WHAT FEELS RIGHT

With a little practice, you will find yourself moving smoothly from one technique to the next as you massage your baby, applying the strokes that feel most comfortable for the area you are working on. The ones described here and on the following page are simply suggestions to get you started. As you try out a variety of strokes, you may find that your baby responds better to some than to others, or you may find that some of them don't come as easily to you. Feel free to leave those out and invent your own – you can try these out on yourself until they feel natural.

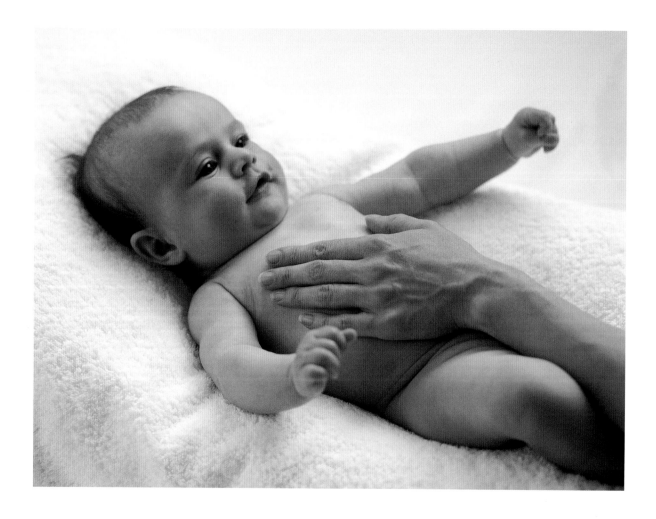

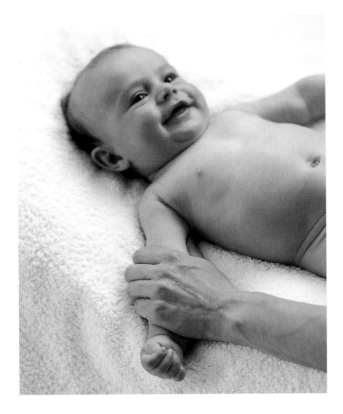

'When I first tried the massage techniques, amazingly my busy boy was calm and still for almost twenty minutes — and we both had a lovely, thoroughly relaxing time.'

KATH, MOTHER OF BEN

DON'T FORGET

Each time you start a massage, remember these points:
□ Your hands should be warm and clean; you will find it easier to do most of the massage strokes if you have reasonably short fingernails.
□ The pressure applied should be firm and not ticklish; babies prefer firm handling and may get restless if they sense hesitancy.
□ Ideally, one of your hands should be kept in constant contact with your baby's skin; it can be disconcerting for the baby to have the massage contact broken. When you reach over to scoop up more oil, or if you need to alter your position slightly, rest your forearm gently on your baby while you do this.

BASIC MASSAGE STROKES

The three basic massage strokes you will use are open-hand technique (also known as drape), closed-hand technique (also known as wrap) and finger strokes.

OPEN-HAND TECHNIQUE

Rest your whole hand across the area, with your fingers relaxed and floppy, as if it were a piece of fabric being draped. Warmth from your palms will relax your baby. Keep your hands soft as you glide them over his skin.

CLOSED-HAND TECHNIQUE

A closed-hand wrap can be very comforting – try this technique when massaging your baby's feet, legs and arms. Slide your hand along the arms or legs, keeping it soft but using a reasonably firm pressure.

FINGER STROKES

Use the soft pads of your fingers to stroke your baby's skin in a grazing motion, without allowing your nails to make contact with the baby's skin. This is a softer massage technique for more delicate areas such as the face or scalp. Finger strokes can be applied more firmly on the back or abdomen.

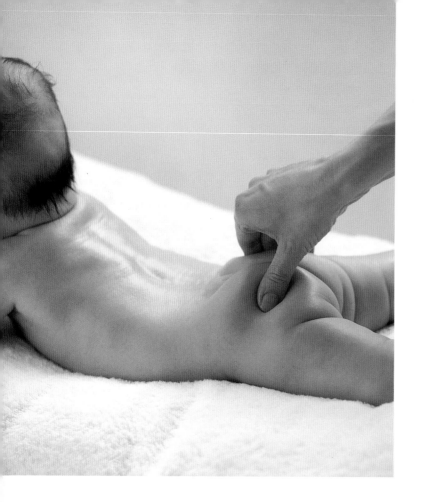

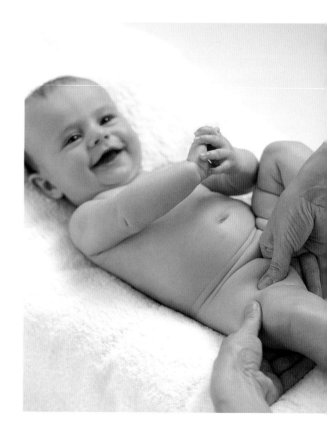

more massage techniques

It is wonderfully rewarding to elicit a sudden chuckle in the middle of a massage – undoubtedly, you and your baby will have favourites among the various techniques, so be guided by what seems to work best for the two of you.

THE RIGHT STROKE FOR THE AREA

The massage techniques illustrated on these pages are shown being used on areas of the body where they might typically be applied. Suggestions for alternative techniques are made in the sections covering massage of specific parts of the body (pages 34–43). Before you start to massage, remember to smooth plenty of oil onto your hands to reduce friction; when this has been absorbed by your baby's skin, add more.

SQUEEZING

Squeezing is a massage technique that is suitable for use on plump fleshy areas such as a baby's thigh or buttock (the gluteus maximus). Squeezing is usually done firmly with the whole hand.

The best method of application is by plenty of short squeezes – it can be very effective to administer little squeezes along your baby's arms to encourage her to 'let go' and relax her elbows.

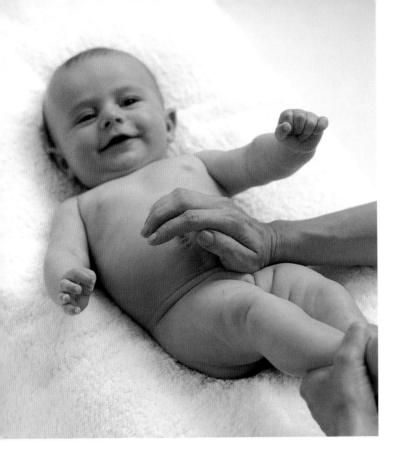

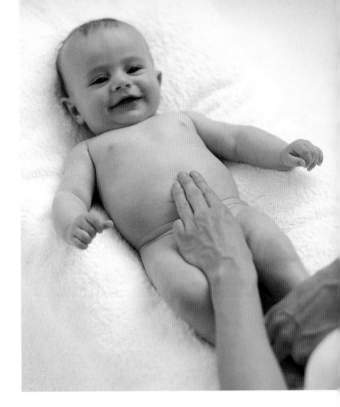

STRETCHING

Tension is released when the skin is gently stretched by opposing thumbs. This can be done firmly on fleshy areas such as thighs, and more gently on a baby's face, where it can be used across the forehead and eyebrows.

KNEADING

Kneading imitates the technique that is used to prepare dough for making bread, with the heel of the hand and then the fingers, in turn. As well as pushing and pulling, there is a slight 'rocking' element to this movement. This stroke can also be done with only the heel of the hand, moving it in a clockwise direction.

CIRCLING

Circling is an appropriate massage technique for the abdomen – using either the whole hand for large circles, or only the fingers for smaller ones. You can also make circles on your baby's scalp, using just enough pressure to move the skin. This circling stroke can be applied with your thumbs around each ankle bone, and on the palms of her hands.

SLIDING

Massage is all about sliding – oil makes possible a firmer pressure than on dry skin, where this technique might be uncomfortable. Slide your fingers along your baby's fingers and toes, for example.

FEATHERING

Feathering is a technique that uses a progressively lighter touch with just the pads of your fingers. It is applied towards the end of the massage, to indicate to your baby that you are gradually withdrawing.

introducing a baby to massage

Since a full-body massage might be overwhelming for a very young baby, introduce massage little by little – and steadily build up your sessions over a period of several weeks to incorporate the full complement of techniques.

KEEP IT GRADUAL

A gradual approach is especially appropriate if you are starting massage with a newborn or very young baby, who may become overstimulated and exhausted by a long session. Give your baby plenty of encouragement by smiling and praising him as you go.

KEEP IT SHORT

Massage has a powerful effect on the central nervous system, so a little goes a long way. When introducing a baby to massage, five minutes is enough to begin with, and massaging only the baby's feet and legs is a good first stage (see pages 34–35).

Each time you massage your baby, make a mental note of how he responds, and build up to longer sessions as he becomes familiar with the sensations.

MASSAGE WITHOUT OIL

Babies frequently complain loudly when being dressed or undressed; if your baby cries when you take off his clothes, one way to accustom him to massage is simply to stroke him over his clothes, to get him used to the feeling. This is also good for very small babies or babies up to three or four weeks old.

Place one hand on his abdomen and move it slowly in circles, in a clockwise direction; hold him against your shoulder while you start gently stroking his back, and finger-stroke the sides of his face and his scalp.

MASSAGE WITH OIL

You can introduce oil for the first time on your baby's feet and legs, without removing any clothing from the rest of his body while you massage. Alternatively, after his bath, place a warm towel across his torso to keep him feeling safe and cosy while you massage oil into his feet and legs.

Warm oil is more liquid and will flow comfortably over his skin without creating any drag. Smooth the oil from his ankle to his thigh and make small circles with your fingers or thumbs.

SKIN CONTACT

Premature babies are known to become calmer if they have skin-to-skin contact with their mothers, and such closeness is also a good introduction to massage. The daily bathtime offers an opportunity for you and your baby to enjoy skin contact and stroking.

When you begin a massage session, touch your baby with more than just your hands – wear a short-sleeved top so that you can sweep your forearms across your baby's chest and abdomen while you stroke his face with your fingertips.

a lovely state of **quiet alertness**, when your baby is **awake, happy and calm**, often follows a massage

LITTLE AND OFTEN

Repetition is the basis of all learning, and repetition is habit-forming. If you settle down in the same place every morning and begin by massaging your baby's feet, he will quickly recognize the new routine. Before long he will respond with pleasure when he sees you begin preparations for his massage.

WORK SLOWLY

Do the strokes very slowly and talk soothingly to your baby, telling him what you are doing and giving him lots of eye contact, smiles and praise. The tempo at which you massage will set the scene for the activity, showing your baby that this is 'downtime' when he can expect uninterrupted attention – his favourite treat.

TRY SOME SOUND EFFECTS

Music can instantly change our mood and induce in us a sense of relaxation, and it will do something similar for most babies. The soothing sounds played to us when we board an aeroplane – designed to reduce heart rate, slow breathing and lower anxiety levels – exemplify the kind of music that will create a calming background for your massage session. Babies also seem to like music with a swing or lilt to it, such as jazz – or why not try singing while you massage?

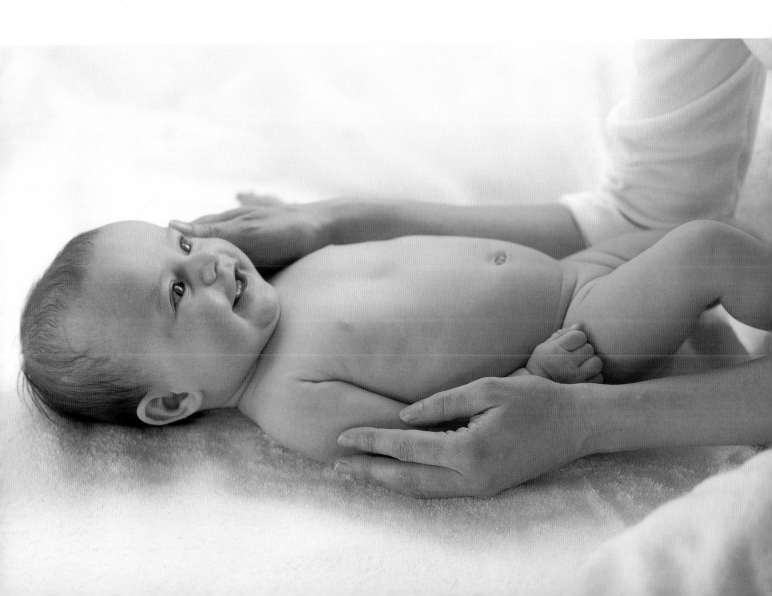

massaging the feet and legs

Perhaps babies like having their feet and legs massaged so much because they can easily watch what is happening; there are hundreds of nerve endings in your baby's feet, which makes them especially responsive to your touch.

THE PERFECT STARTING POINT

Rare is the baby who does not like having feet and legs massaged, which makes this area the perfect starting point. Engage your baby's attention, smile and explain what you are doing and why. It is this interaction that babies love, because it signals that you are doing this activity with them, not to them. Babies often have cold hands and feet; if this is the case, your touch will immediately start to warm the baby, and you can give little squeezes to improve the circulation.

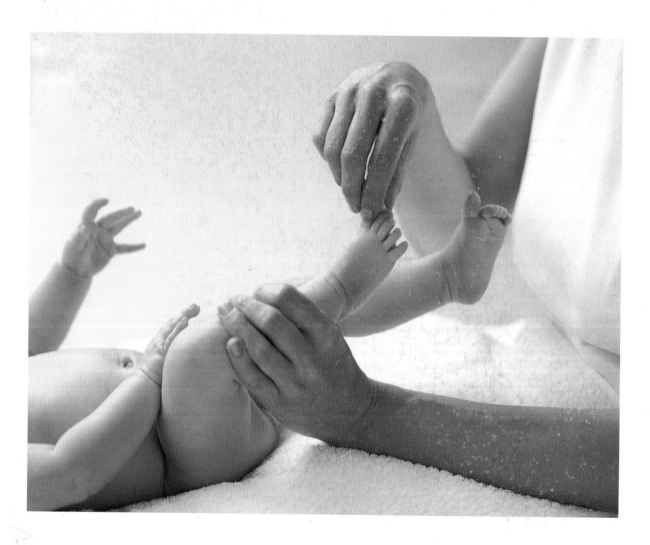

THE SEQUENCE

step 1

To begin the massage, scoop up some oil, rubbing it between your hands to warm it, and simply wrap each hand around your baby's feet.

step 2

Slide your baby's feet through your hands over and over again until her feet have warmed up. Then stroke your fingers along each toe in turn.

step 3

Take hold of her right ankle in your right hand, raising her right leg in the air. Wrap your other hand around her leg and slide your hand down from ankle to thigh; you can also slide from thigh back to ankle. The first is Swedish massage, which strokes towards the heart to improve circulation; the second is Indian massage, which strokes away from the centre, for relaxation. Repeat on the left leg.

step 4

Still holding your baby's ankle with one hand, enclose her calf muscle with the other hand and give it a few squeezes. As long as you apply plenty of oil, your hand will slip off as you do this, making it impossible to squeeze too hard.

step 5

Take hold of your baby's thigh with one or both hands, and make circles with your thumbs all over the area. This fleshy area is the ideal place for baby massage.

step 6

When you have massaged each of your baby's thighs in turn, wrap your hands around both legs and continue to squeeze and press.

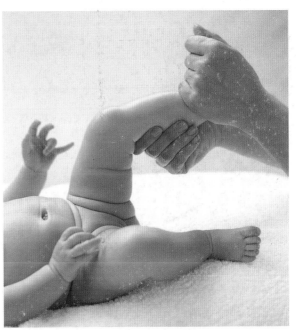

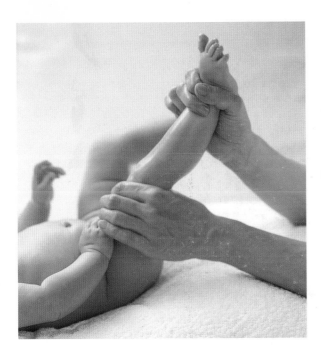

massaging the abdomen and chest

There are many therapeutic benefits from massaging the abdomen and chest, but remember to massage slowly, and if your baby cries at first simply try again later. It is a good idea to wait for at least 15 minutes after a feed.

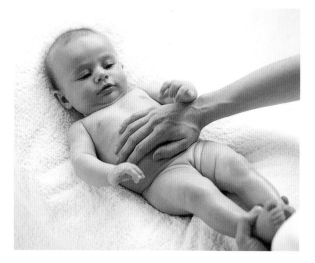

TAKE IT GRADUALLY

Babies can be a little uncertain at first about being massaged on the abdomen. It is the centre of a great deal of important activity, and, no doubt, many different sensations. Introduce massage in this area very gradually, by simply resting one hand across the abdomen without moving, allowing the warmth of your palm to reach your baby's skin before you continue.

Don't worry if your baby struggles or cries when you first massage her abdomen. It can take a few attempts and a gradual approach for some babies to accept massage here; try again on another occasion.

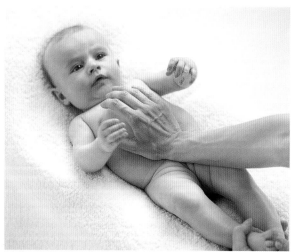

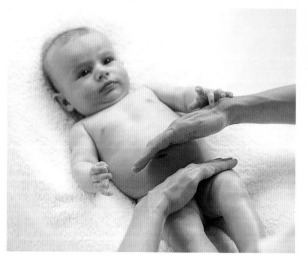

to **reassure** a doubtful baby, start by simply resting

one hand across the abdomen **without moving**

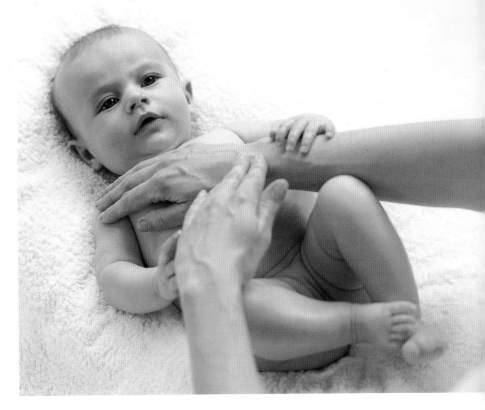

'He loves the massage now, and it has helped to settle a very restless, colicky baby.'

CYNTHIA, MOTHER OF BENJAMIN

THE SEQUENCE

step 1

With a relaxed, open hand and using plenty of oil, stroke your baby's abdomen slowly in clockwise circles, avoiding the umbilical cord area until it has fully healed. You can also massage in smaller circles all around this area with the pads of your fingers.

Massaging in a clockwise direction follows the path of the colon, easing digestive troubles such as wind and colic. For constipation, massage once or twice in the reverse direction, and then clockwise a few more times. The following strokes particularly help in relieving wind.

step 2

Position your hand just below the navel and, kneading with the heel of your hand, make circles in a clockwise direction. You can also knead from side to side, below the rib cage, alternately pushing with the heel of your hand and then pulling back with your fingers.

step 3

Use a 'paddling' stroke downwards over your baby's abdomen, with one hand following the other in a scooping movement. This is called the Waterwheel.

step 4

To finish, massage your baby's chest with open-hand crossover strokes. Start at the shoulders and stroke diagonally across her chest with each hand in turn. Follow this by moving both your hands together up the chest and along the arms. Chest massage helps to improve lung function.

'I didn't think Evie would lie still because she's very active, like me. But I find doing the massage makes me relax so she picks up on that and does the same.'

CAROL, MOTHER OF EVIE

massaging the arms and hands

Babies are very busy with their arms and hands, and may not want to let you massage both at once – take every opportunity to stroke and massage them whenever you are having a cuddle with your baby.

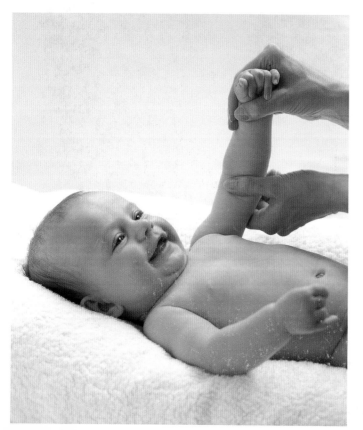

ONE ARM AT A TIME

Babies commonly show their enjoyment by wriggling about and waving their arms and legs. They may seem to resist when you attempt to hold both their arms at the same time – in which case, massage each of the arms individually, leaving the baby with the other one free while you do so.

STRAIGHTENING OUT

Since it is instinctive for your baby to keep the elbows bent and held tightly into the body, it may be difficult to get the baby to straighten out the arms for massage. Babies vary in the age at which they let go of this protective pose. If your baby holds her arms tightly into her body, simply stroke down the outsides of the arms, until she is ready to relax.

THE SEQUENCE

step 1

Take one of your baby's wrists in one of your hands, then slide your other hand along her arm from wrist to shoulder, in the same way as you did with her legs (see pages 34–35). Repeat this stroke on the other arm. Then, still holding her at the wrist, use your other hand to thumb press all along her arm or squeeze with your thumb and fingers.

step 2

Try wrapping both your hands around your baby's arms at the shoulders and stroking down to the hands. If your baby is very active, include some small squeezes to encourage her to relax her arms. See if you can coax her to open her arms out wide.

step 3

You can stroke across the back of her hands using your fingers, and then, if your baby's fingers are starting to uncurl, stroke the palm of your hand across the palm of your baby's hand. Slide along each of her fingers in turn, holding them up so she can watch.

step 4

Stroke your thumbs in small circles in the palms of your baby's hands.

step 5

Hold her hands (or wrists) and open her arms wide, then cross them over her chest in a 'hug'. Repeat this if your baby enjoys it – the stretch will help to open her airways and exercise her back and shoulder muscles.

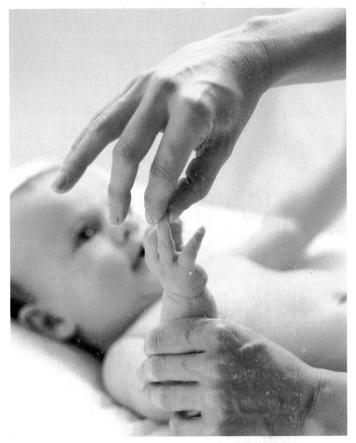

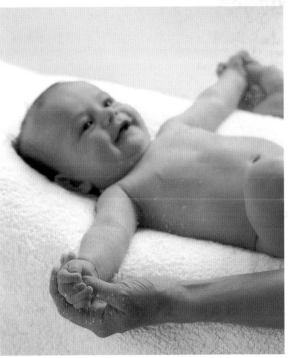

massaging the head and face

Massaging your baby's head and face can ease teething pain, clear a blocked nose, relieve and prevent colds, and encourage sleep. Only a short massage is necessary, with a lighter touch on the skin of your baby's face.

NATURAL LUBRICATION

Your baby's face has its own natural oil, so there is no need to apply oil when you massage the head and face. Wipe off any excess oil from your fingers before you start, and try to keep any oil away from your baby's eyes – she may rub an oily hand into her eyelid, so have a tissue ready. When oil may come into contact with a baby's face, it is safest to use an edible, unscented kind.

Face massage is most effective when you lean in close and maintain eye contact. Perform these strokes gently but firmly, and smile to hold your baby's attention.

THE SEQUENCE

step 1

Begin with an open-hand stroke to massage the sides of your baby's head, avoiding the delicate fontanelle on

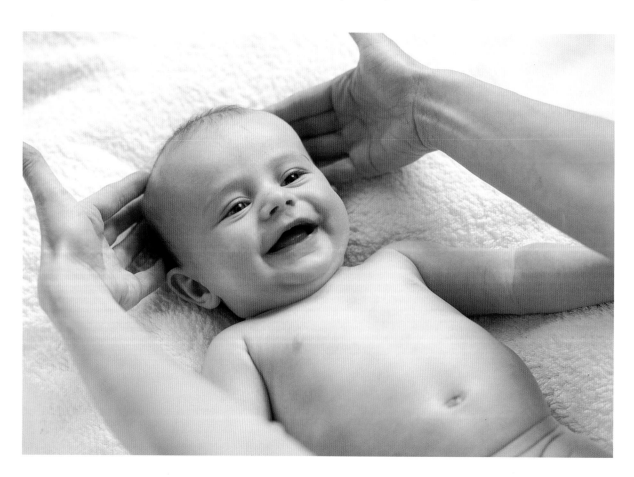

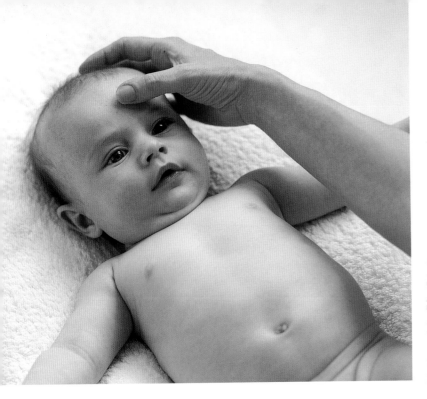

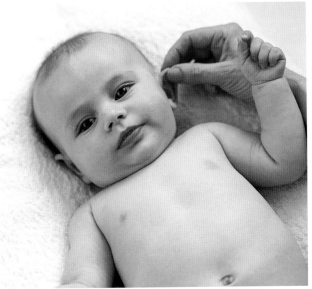

top. Use a little oil to relieve cradlecap, eczema or dry skin on the scalp. Relax your hands as you massage the head with wide sweeping strokes, then massage her scalp with your fingers in small circular strokes.

step 2
Cradle her head in your fingers (see opposite) while you stroke and stretch across the brow with your thumbs. Continue the same stretching stroke down each side of the nose and across the cheekbones, using a firm pressure. These are the sinus areas, where massage can help to relieve congestion and clear your baby's nose.

step 3
Use the same technique to stroke and stretch above and below your baby's lips, and under her chin. Follow this by massaging all over her cheeks with the pads of your fingers. When your baby is teething you can massage inside her mouth with your finger along the lower gum, where the first two teeth will emerge.

step 4
Use your thumbs to uncurl the outside edge of the ears, and stroke a dab of oil behind the ear lobe, where there is often a patch of dry skin.

step 5
A soothing finishing touch is a thumb stroke down from the hairline to a point between the eyebrows. When your baby is drowsy or wakes at night, you can coax her back to sleep with this stroke – referred to in Chinese baby massage as 'closing the head door'.

babies seem to love the feeling of having **little tufts** of their hair **gently tweaked**, which stimulates the whole scalp

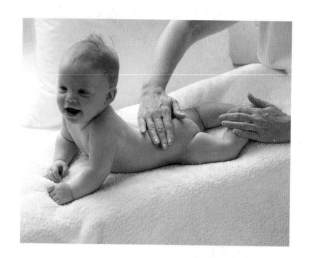

'The twins really enjoyed
having their backs massaged.
They were so relaxed and happy
afterwards — and very sleepy.'

TRACEY, MOTHER OF HOPE AND MILES

massaging the back and spine

Three alternative positions for back massage are suggested here. When massaging the back, stroking downwards from the neck is considered to be soothing and calming, while stroking upwards is stimulating and invigorating. You can choose either or both.

POSITION 1: LYING SIDEWAYS

A young baby will feel comfortable lying across your lap, with your hand holding his shoulder and your arm supporting his chest. His head may droop down or turn sideways to rest on your arm.

POSITION 2: SITTING

A sitting position suits a young baby, who can lean slightly forwards, using your arm for support, while you massage his back. Older babies may like to sit up while having their backs massaged – or try the position using a cushion described in Becoming Mobile (pages 48–49).

POSITION 3: LYING LENGTHWAYS

When your baby has developed enough strength in his neck muscles to hold up his head without support, usually at the age of around four months, he can lie lengthways on his front for massage. This is the ideal position because it allows you to use both your hands for the massage. It is also quite tiring for your baby, so

he may eventually put his head down to rest, but don't let him fall asleep in this position; for safety's sake, babies should always be put to sleep on their backs.

THE SEQUENCE

step 1

Using one or both hands, massage in one smooth stroke from the back of your baby's head right down to his feet. Repeat this stroke many times, keeping it firm and slow. You can also stroke from side to side, with your hands crossing the baby's back in turn.

step 2

Place one hand at your baby's neck and the other on his feet; slide your hands together to give the big muscles in his buttocks a squeeze.

step 3

Finish the massage with some gentler strokes, known as feathering, to show your baby the massage is ending.

BABY MASSAGE

42

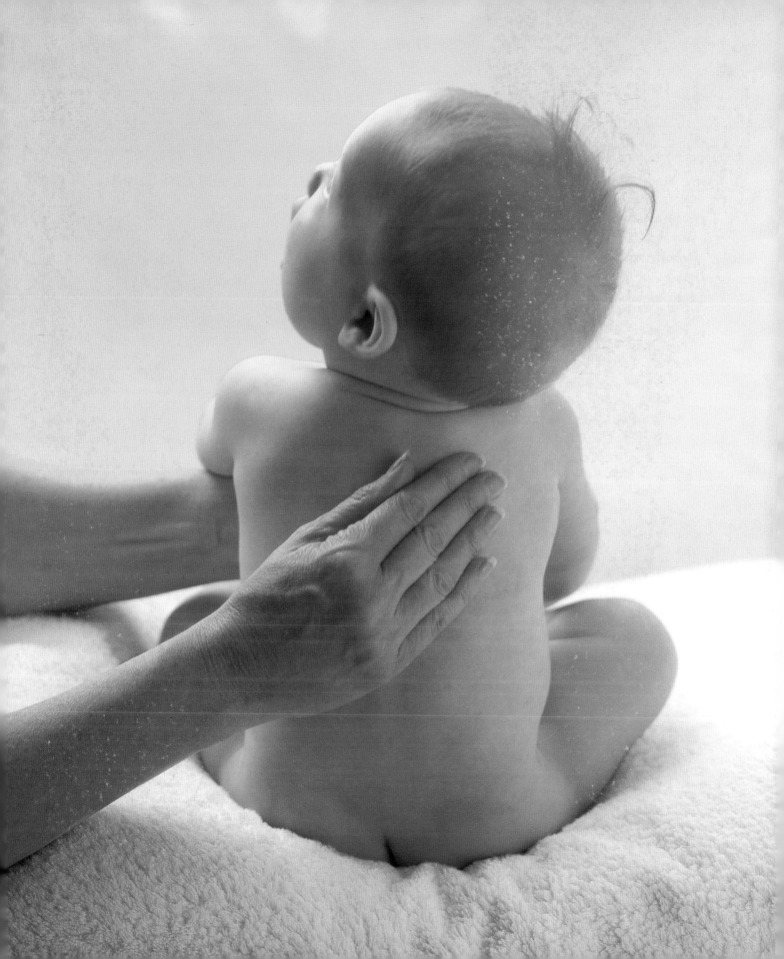

Learning the techniques is only part of the story of baby massage. As well as touch, add your favourite sounds and aromas to delight the senses. Success is about creating an intimate atmosphere that makes the experience special.

TEN WAYS TO... *succeed at massage*

1 Massage is stimulating, and your baby should be fully awake and ready to play when you begin. You may find the best time is in the morning after a nap or bath. A tired baby cannot be massaged to sleep and will only get cross and cranky if you try.

2 To respond well to massage, your baby needs to be toasty warm: the room should be around 26°C (80°F) or a little cooler if your baby has eczema. Warm the oil, either by rubbing it between your hands before you apply it or by warming a bowl before adding oil.

3 Make sure you have some drinks to hand for you both. Massage in a warm room can be thirsty work, and dehydration makes you feel tired. Your baby may want to stop for some refreshment during the session, so take the opportunity to drink a glass of water or fruit juice for instant revival.

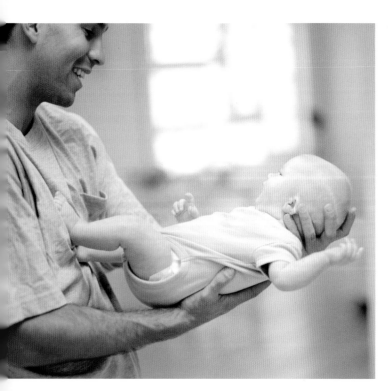

4 Babies relax when their mothers relax! Play your favourite 'unwinding' CD while you gather what you need and prepare the room. Before sitting down, hold your baby close and sway to the music for a while to get rid of tension in your hips, back and shoulders.

5 By four months of age your baby will enjoy holding and playing with a toy while you massage her; have a basket of small toys nearby and give her one at a time, replacing it with another when she loses interest.

6 Adjusting curtains or blinds to create a shaded, more intimate atmosphere will help you to 'tune in' to your sense of touch and make it easier to maintain eye contact with your baby.

7 Unlike adults, babies like lots of entertainment while being massaged. It can be fun to meet up with a friend so you can massage your babies together – from the age of five months or so, your baby will start to notice and show an interest in other babies.

8 Remind yourself that massage rewards the person giving it as well as the one receiving with a calmer heart rate and a burst of feel-good hormones.

9 If your baby starts to get fussy during massage, she may simply want to be moved to a new position. If you know that she doesn't need to feed or sleep, lifting her up for a quick change of viewpoint often does the trick, and then you can resume the massage.

10 Forget about schedules. At the best of times babies are unpredictable; some days you will find that your baby will accept a longer massage, and on other days just five or ten minutes will be enough. Let yourself be guided by what she wants. Even a short massage will have a very beneficial effect.

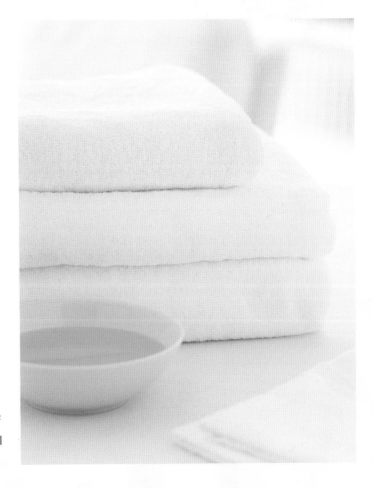

techniques to encourage good posture

We marvel at the flexibility of babies and toddlers, but this can be lost as they grow and develop poor postural habits. Safeguard your baby's future mobility by encouraging these stretching and strengthening poses.

POSTURAL DEVELOPMENT

When you watch your baby effortlessly put his toes into his mouth, it is easy to imagine that he will stay as flexible as he is now for years to come. But he is more vulnerable to postural damage than you may realize. Such damage – which is commonly caused by sitting on poorly designed chairs at school and being obliged to remain immobile for long periods – is seen in children as young as seven. This is despite the fact that young children instinctively choose correct posture – for example, by tipping a chair forward so that it balances on two legs, a child's knees will be lower than his hips, resulting in a straight spine. This echoes the principle of the orthopaedic 'back chair', which incorporates knee support below the seat.

Poor posture affects more than just the spine; it compresses the abdomen and internal organs and leads to digestive and breathing problems. However, there are a variety of ways in which you can help your baby to develop a strong back and lay the foundation for good posture for the future.

LYING AND SITTING

Don't leave your baby in a car seat once you have finished a journey, as tempting as it may be to let him take a nap there. Babies need to lie flat as much as possible until they can sit up unaided, at the age of around six months.

When you do sit your baby up, give him seats with proper back support to encourage a good upright sitting posture. Non-rigid baby seats and buggies that leave your baby neither sitting nor lying flat are doing your child no favours – watch how a toddler will struggle to 'sit up' in one of these. It is the equivalent of lying in a hammock – less comfortable than it looks.

MUSCLE DEVELOPMENT

From the age of three to four months, it is important to lie your baby on his front for a short time every day so that he can develop the muscles needed to hold up his head. Even if, at first, your baby does not like lying on his front, encourage him with reassurances and by making it enjoyable. You will be surprised how quickly your baby's neck muscles will strengthen. Place his arms in front of him so that he can use them for support. This position also strengthens the back – by six months of age, he will be able to rock back and forth with his arms and legs off the floor.

FLEXIBILITY

Baby massage sessions can include various stretching and bending exercises such as the hug described on page 39. Your baby's legs can be crossed over in a way similar to the arm movement used in the hug: make sure that his knees are bent and the movement is done slowly and without force. You can then cross one arm with the opposite leg, and repeat on the other side.

Older babies love to do forward and backward bends. Before your baby can do these independently, you can encourage the movements by supporting his head while you help him to lean as far forward or back as he wants to. Both of these stretches help to increase flexibility of the spine.

CRAWLING

Even when your baby is no more than a few weeks old, you can do 'pedalling' movements with his legs while

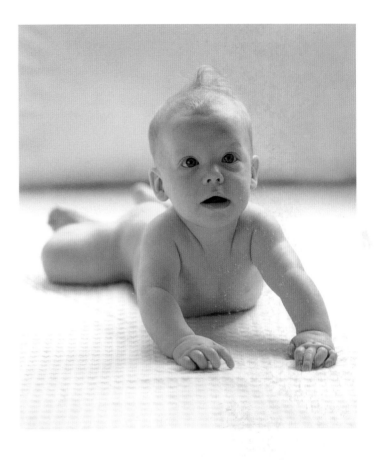

he lies on his back – vary the speed from slow and deliberate to faster and more energetic to keep his interest. This will encourage crawling when he reaches that stage. Crawling plays a role in the development of the spine, according to teachers of the Alexander Technique, who recommend rocking gently back and forth on all fours to relieve a bad back. You can encourage your baby to do this by getting down on the floor with him and doing it too.

exercised babies tend to cry less and **sleep better**, so it works wonders to include in your massage routine a few **simple stretches** to add **energy** and **fun**

becoming mobile

From six months onwards, massage is more active and vigorous to keep pace with your baby's increasing mobility and to help muscle growth; later on, your toddler can be soothed and calmed with her favourite strokes.

UP AND AWAY

Almost before you know it, your baby will be on the move. One day you will turn around and she will have discovered how to roll over onto her front – and from there it will seem a matter of moments before she is up and away. But, some time before that day arrives, you are likely to find that your baby will no longer want to lie on her back for a long period while you give her a massage. There is no need to give up on massage – simply try some new positions that allow her to look around, hold and play with a toy, or perhaps to interact with someone else in the room.

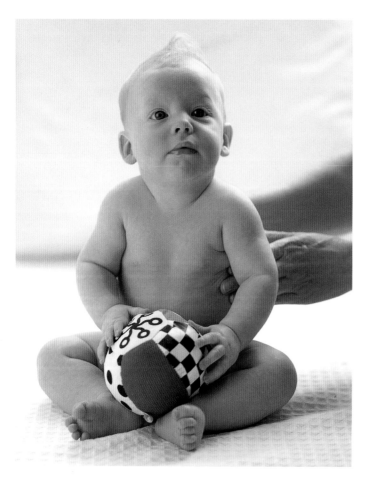

MASSAGE POSITIONS

One idea is simply to sit up your baby in your lap, with her back against your front. Do this close to a mirror (or prop up a mirror nearby) so that you can still see each other's face. It doesn't matter if you don't do all the massage strokes: be inventive and adapt them to suit the new circumstances. From this position, for example, you can easily stroke and squeeze the back of her neck and massage her shoulders.

Another position suitable for a more mobile baby is to sit her up and allow her to lean forward to rest on a medium-sized cushion while you massage her back. To keep her occupied while you are massaging, place a toy or baby book within her reach, and talk to her.

MASSAGE FROM SIX MONTHS TO ONE YEAR

Your baby may have outgrown colic by six months but can still benefit from massage at this stage. Demanding new activities can lead to over-stimulation and a restless baby who won't sleep. A daytime massage will reduce stress levels and lead to deeper sleep later on.

While generally uncommon in babies, constipation can follow the introduction of solid foods; this can easily be relieved by a circular massage of the abdomen or the kneading strokes outlined on pages 31 and 37.

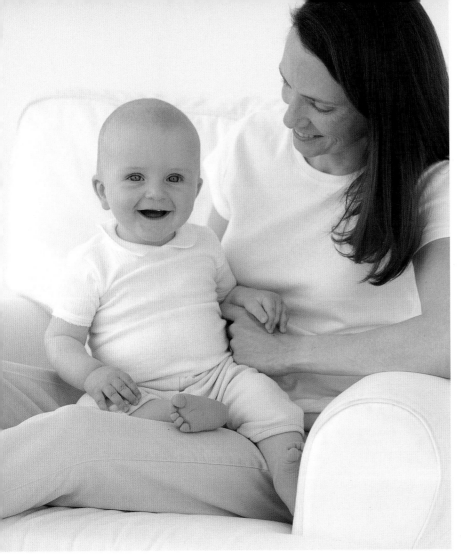

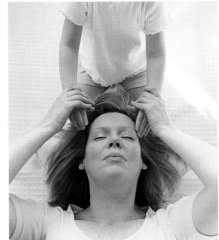

Regularly massaged babies demonstrate a reduced stress response to inoculations at the age of one year, and better physical coordination and confidence than others in their age group.

TODDLER MASSAGE

Massage with a toddler can be a challenge, requiring patience and good humour on the parent's part. As with babies, however, a regular massage will be easier if it has the same associations each time; give your toddler a selection of CDs to choose from before you start, and perhaps have a special towel that you always use for massage. Helping to get these things ready will put her in a cooperative frame of mind.

BEING NEEDED

One thing all toddlers respond to is the feeling of being needed, so ask your child if she will massage you first. She can stroke your face and head, then you can massage each other's feet and hands. To avoid spills, you could use a nicely scented handcream from a tube instead of oil. If you have a baby as well, your toddler can be given a doll and some oil in a bowl, so that she can copy you as you massage the baby.

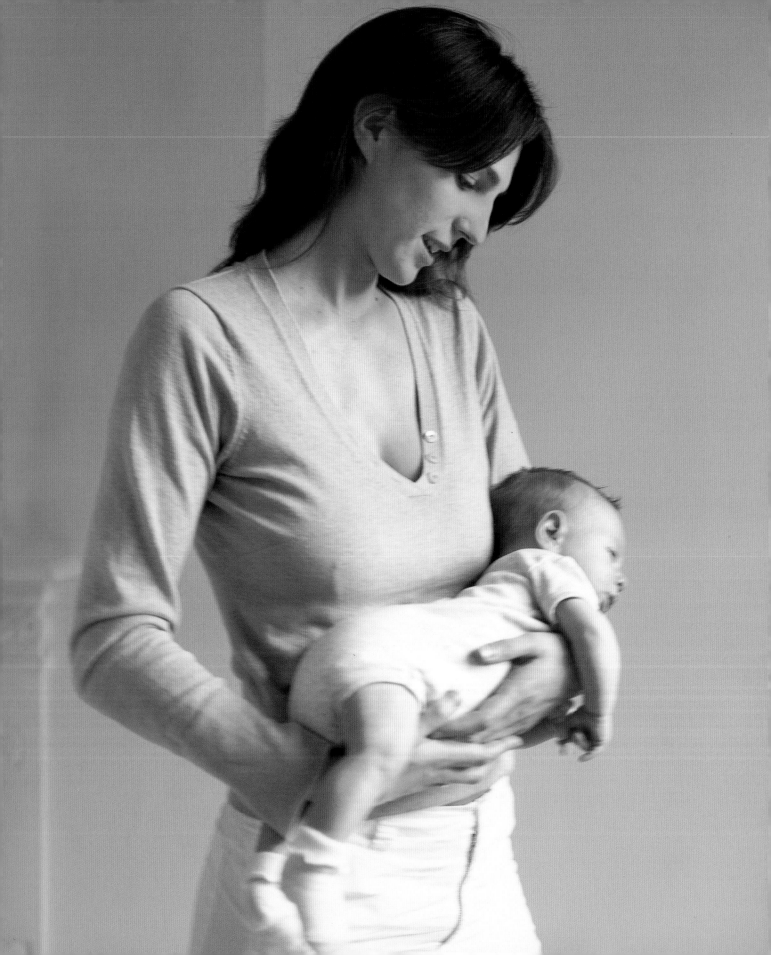

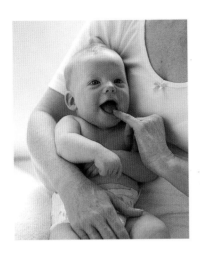

your questions answered

Regular massage will enhance your baby's physical and emotional health and well-being, while specific strokes can help to relieve common baby ailments.

CAN IT BE HARMFUL TO MASSAGE A BABY?

Baby massage is generally safe but there are some times when it is inadvisable – for example, when your baby has a raised temperature or seems otherwise unwell, including just after immunization. Don't massage if your baby has recently had surgery or is lethargic, and avoid massaging where there is infection or skin damage or over the area of an immunization. Overstimulation can prevent sleep, so don't massage when the baby is tired.

HOW LONG SHOULD I MASSAGE MY BABY, AND HOW FREQUENTLY?

Your baby will get the most benefit from massage if you make it part of his playtime routine, either daily, if you can, or three to four times a week. Be guided by your baby as to how long the session should last. A 20 minute session is generally about right, but anything from ten minutes to half an hour or longer is fine. He will definitely let you know when he is ready to stop!

WILL MASSAGE HELP MY BABY TO SLEEP?

Regular massage will improve your baby's sleep pattern and help him to fall asleep more quickly; however, massage stimulates the nervous system so your baby will not necessarily fall asleep straight after a massage. It is the frequency of massage, rather than the timing, which helps with sleep, so always massage your baby when he is wide awake, not when he is tired.

IS THERE ANYTHING I CAN DO FOR TEETHING?

When your baby starts teething, you can massage all around his jaw line with your fingertips. You can also rub your finger along his gums where the teeth are coming through. First, dip your finger in lemon juice, which has anti-inflammatory properties.

MY BABY HAS ECZEMA – IS IT SAFE TO USE OIL?

Natural oils are perfectly safe, but carry out an allergy test if you are using oil for the first time (see page 25). Massage can help to relax your baby and relieve itching. With eczema, towel fibres can tickle and irritate, so lay your baby on a smooth cotton surface for massage.

CAN MASSAGE RELIEVE COLIC?

Massaging the abdomen briefly has been found to ease colic. Another remedy is the position shown opposite (known variously as Tiger in a Tree, the football hold or the rugby hold), which often has a soothing effect. This may be because it puts pressure on the abdomen while allowing the baby some freedom to move. Gently rock and shush your baby in this position.

CAN I MASSAGE MY BABY IF HE HAS A COLD?

If your baby has a cold you should not undress him for a massage, but you can help clear a blocked nose by stroking your thumbs down the sides of his nose and following the strokes for the sinus areas (see page 41).

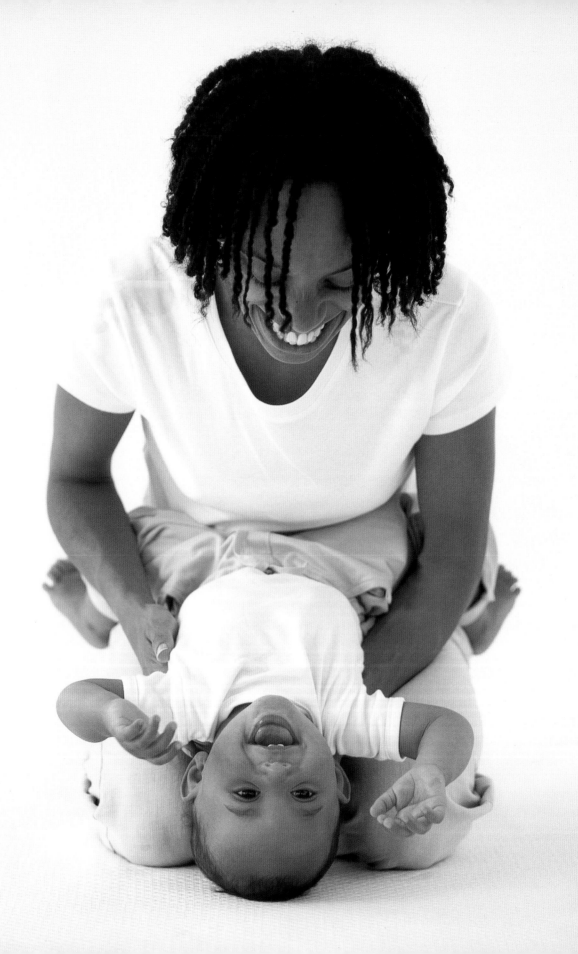

baby yoga and gym

Babies have a natural aptitude for yoga and gym. Their newly uncurled bodies are ready to stretch and open out to the experience of the world around them. Reflecting a gentle progression from baby massage, yoga and gym also stimulate loving interaction between parent and child – a fulfilling and rewarding experience for you both.

yoga and gym: the principles

Baby yoga and gym involve postures, stretches and exercises that you can do with your child to promote healthy development; they also offer you a way to be supportive and encouraging to your child at every stage. You may prefer to try some of the movements for the first time in the context of a baby yoga class.

A CONTINUING JOY

The aim of baby yoga and gym is to promote health in babies and children by means of postures, exercises and stretches through movement. Yoga and gym also offer you a way to be attentive to your child's needs and to encourage your child's fast development.

Baby yoga and gym are a natural progression from massage, which is good preparation for the postures and movements. You can introduce your baby to yoga from the age of two to three months (see pages 56–69). When babies begin to crawl and become more active, they are less likely to keep still, so this is a good time to begin baby gym (see pages 70–79). At this stage your child is more mobile, stronger and better coordinated, and will enjoy being handled a little more vigorously.

Years of teaching baby massage, yoga and gym have allowed me to observe the physical and psychological growth and development of my two sons and that of many other children. I have seen their confidence increase, their bodies become strong and supple, and their keen sense of adventure nurtured. It has been a continuing joy to see the children engage in these activities with such uninhibited enthusiasm.

BE GUIDED BY YOUR CHILD

Baby yoga postures and baby gym movements should progress in line with natural physical development. Rather than thinking that children should be doing certain things at certain stages, it is important to be guided by where they are in terms of ability. They are developing at a rate and pace that is right for them. This is a journey of exploration and learning for you and your child, and when family and friends join in, it can be an even more enriching and rewarding experience.

REGULAR PRACTICE

Yoga and gym are excellent ways for children to expend their abundant energy and can be used as creative tools to encourage development. Regular practice of the movements also offers the following benefits.

☐ It strengthens the bond between you and your child.
☐ It increases your confidence in handling your child.
☐ It increases your child's trust in your ability to handle him or her.
☐ It helps to maintain flexibility and suppleness of joints while strengthening the body.
☐ It encourages good coordination of movements, as well as fluidity and agility.
☐ It creates good postural habits.
☐ It strengthens and tones muscles.
☐ It reduces physical tension.

DOS AND DON'TS OF BABY YOGA AND GYM

DO make sure your baby is content and settled.
DO make sure the room you are in is free of obstacles.
DO be safe; you may wish to put mats or cushions on the floor for soft landings for some of the movements.
DO stop and settle a child who cries during the postures or movements. It may be that your child doesn't enjoy a particular movement or is hungry or tired. Once your

child has regained a calm mood, you can return to the exercise – unless your child has lost interest, in which case stop and try it again another day.

DO build up the postures and movements gradually – and have fun in the process.

DON'T do postures or movements if you child is tired or unwell, has just eaten or does not want to do them.

DON'T wear jewellery or clothing that could get in the way of the postures or movements; do all you can to avoid accidents and injuries.

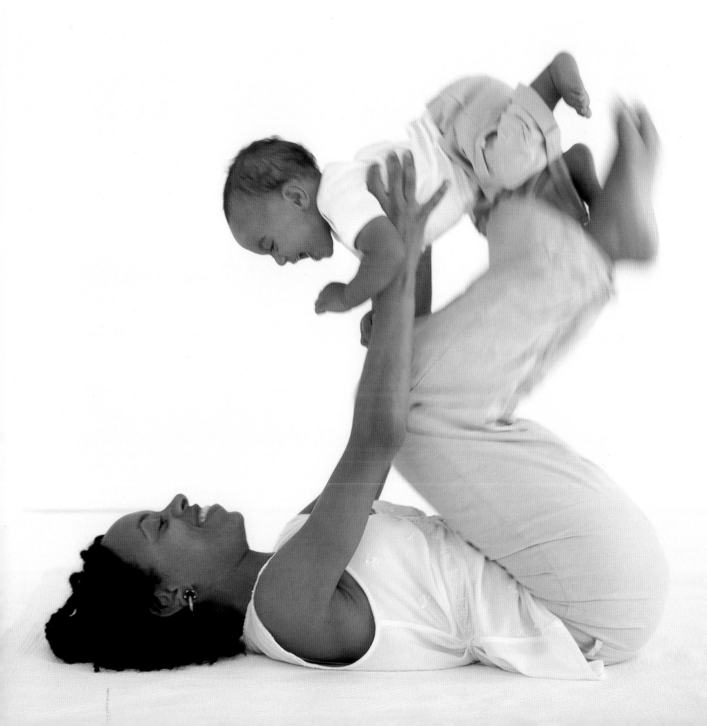

yoga and gym can be separate **activities** or can be done
together and combined with a **massage** routine

tailor pose

This simple pose encourages a correct sitting posture, which is
beneficial for the development of a baby's spine. It also provides
a starting position from which other movements can be made.

WHEN TO START

A good age to introduce a baby to Tailor Pose is three
to four months. By that time, babies should be able to
support the weight of their head, and their muscles
should have developed enough strength and tone to
allow them to keep themselves upright with your aid.

GETTING READY

Sit on the floor with your legs stretched out in side
splits (see page 64) or bend your legs and sit on your
heels. Sit your baby on the floor between your legs and
put your arms under her armpits. Your arms act like a
harness as you pull them in to keep your baby upright.

THE SEQUENCE

step 1

With both hands holding your baby's ankles, bring
the soles of her feet together close to the base of the
spine. Lean her forwards so that her arms are reaching
towards the floor. In time, if she doesn't already do so,
your baby will stretch out her hands on the floor in
front of her for support.

step 2

Place one hand on your baby's chest for support and
stroke down her spine firmly from the top to the base.
Maintain a small pressure at the base. This helps to
'root' the spine and gives your baby added stability
and support while sitting. As you root the spine, you
may notice that your baby is able to support her head
for longer than usual.

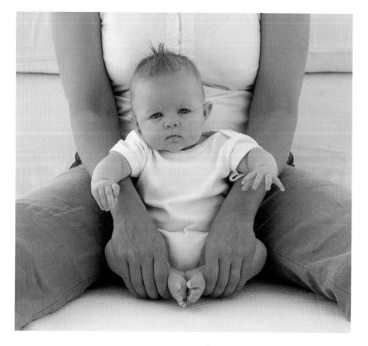

tailor pose swing

Lifting up your baby in Tailor Pose and swinging him gently from side to side adds a new dimension to the idea of fun in motion.

THE SEQUENCE

step 1

Sitting on your heels, with your baby in Tailor Pose on your lap, lift yourself up onto your knees and stand up, supporting your baby with your arms. This movement should feel comfortable for you, and you should take care not to strain your shoulders or back. When you are standing, lean your baby forwards a little, making sure that you keep his feet in line with his hips.

step 2

When you are sure that you have your baby securely held, swing him gently from side to side. Then bring him back down onto your lap in Tailor Pose.

'Since doing Tailor Pose Swing, Kiki has gained strength and can increasingly hold herself up. And she really loves it — she giggles when she sees herself in a mirror.'

VICKI, MOTHER OF KIKI

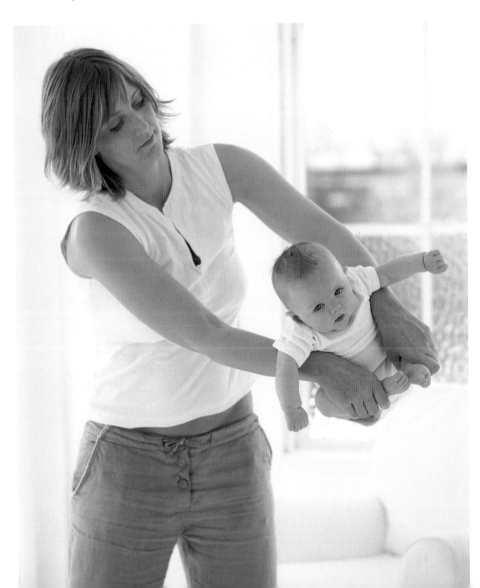

back bend

This exercise stretches the arms and legs and facilitates deep breathing. It also helps your child to uncurl from the foetal position she maintained inside the womb. As long as your baby is happy, repeat the sequence several times.

GETTING READY

Kneel on the floor with your legs together or sit in a chair. Lie your baby across your lap on her back, holding her nearside forearm in your hand.

Encourage her to have a good stretch by patting her chest and saying, 'Aaaaaahhhh.' Babies generally tend to like this, and will gradually build up the confidence to let their head and arms go back and allow their legs to stretch out away from the body.

THE SEQUENCE

step 1

To coax your baby to lie back, stroke your hand across the front of her body so that she can open out, and allow her head to rest on your lap. At first you may be tempted to hold your baby's head for support – or she may want to raise it up.

step 2

Take hold of one leg and the wrist and hand of the opposing arm. Pull on each very gently at the same time, giving her a good stretch along the whole body.

step 3

Repeat the stretch with the other arm and leg.

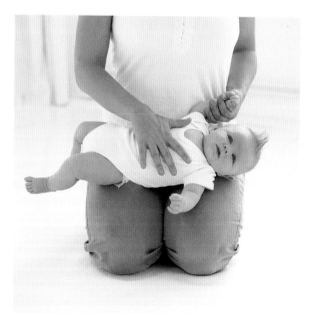

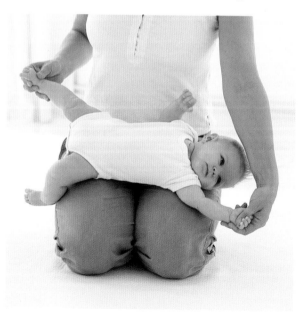

shoulder stand, handstand & hang

This is a good exercise for stretching and relieving tension in the spine. Before trying an upside-down hang, be sure that your baby has developed enough upper-body strength to be able to hold up her own head – and always hold her legs around the shins and calves, not the ankles.

THE SEQUENCE

step 1

This sequence of movements starts with the baby in the Back Bend position, as described opposite.

step 2

For Shoulder Stand, hold your baby around the shins and calves and lift her so she is upside down. To reassure the baby, maintain the contact between her shoulders and your legs, then lie her back down on your lap.

step 3

Once you are confident with Shoulder Stand, and your baby is enjoying it, lift her so that her hands are in contact with your lap and let her relish the experience.

step 4

If your baby is happy, lift her higher so she is no longer touching you. Let her simply hang. You will notice that she flexes her body, taking some of her own weight. After a few moments, lower her gently onto your lap.

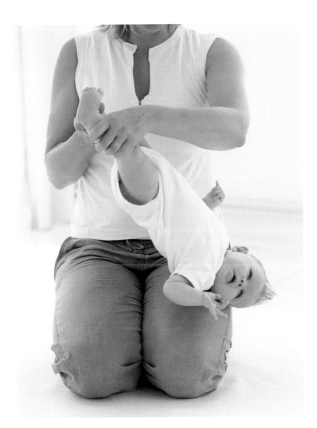
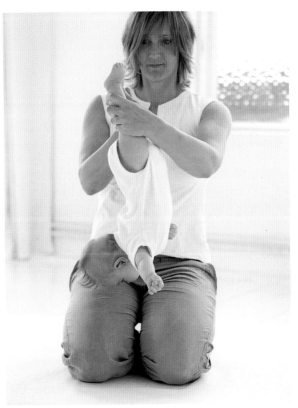

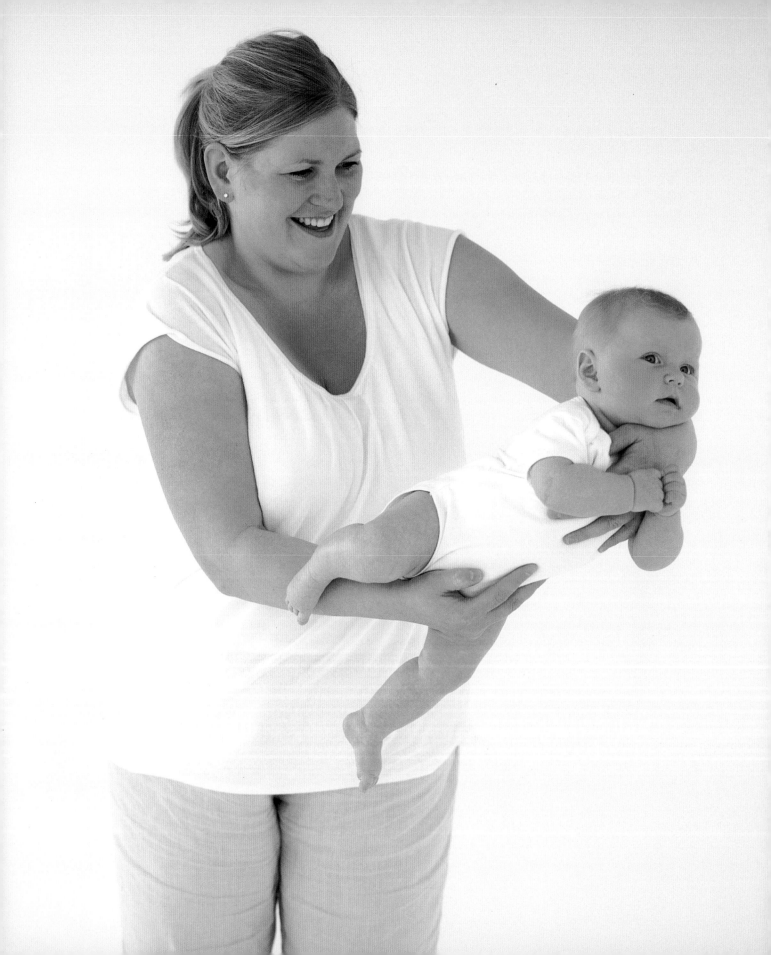

tiger in a tree swing

This is a good position for relieving colic, constipation and trapped wind. The light pressure of your hand over your child's belly will give her some relief – and massaging her in this position will help even more.

SWING OR NO SWING

This sequence involves swinging your baby back and forth, first on her tummy, then on her back, but Tiger in a Tree without the swing is a great position for holding your baby whether or not she has digestive problems. You can also use it for carrying your baby, since it minimizes strain on your back, neck and shoulders.

THE SEQUENCE

step 1

Feed one of your arms up through your baby's legs and place your hand over her belly. Support her around the upper chest with your other hand, allowing her head to rest comfortably on your forearm.

step 2

Swing your child back and forth, continuing with this rocking motion for as long as she remains happy.

step 3

For a change, hold your baby in a similar position on her back. While swinging her back and forth, as before, you can engage with her more intensely by talking, laughing and maintaining eye contact.

'When we first began baby yoga, I was a bit tentative about some of the moves and not very confident. Now we do Tiger in a Tree Swing every day and Loxie is fearless and loves it!'

ANNA, MOTHER OF LOXIE

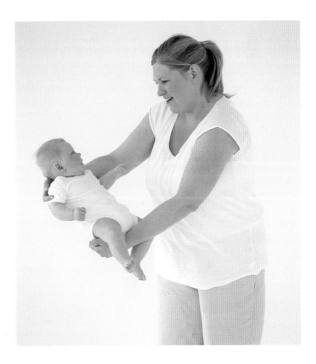

high lift

This exercise will build your baby's confidence and her trust in you as you offer her the opportunity to experience the space around her.

GETTING READY

Your own stance and posture are especially important when doing this exercise: stand with your feet hip-width apart and knees slightly bent. The lift will allow you to give your own back, arms and shoulders a good stretch – but don't do it if you have a back problem.

THE SEQUENCE

step 1

With your baby facing away from you, hold her under her arms and lift her out in front of you. You could sing a nursery rhyme such as 'The Grand Old Duke of York'.

step 2

Making sure your baby knows you have her securely supported, raise her above your head and then lower her back down in front of you. Repeat the lift a few times, until she has had enough.

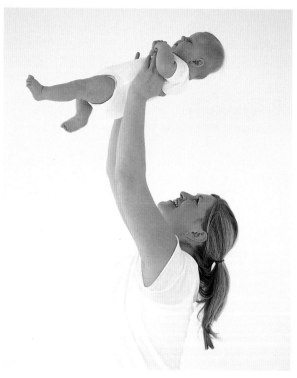

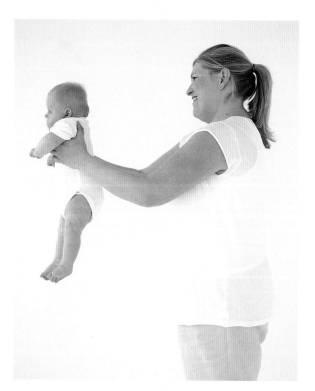

forward bend

This movement goes with the nursery rhyme 'Row Your Boat'. Singing the song at the same time as doing the exercise will help you to guide your child into a forward bend.

ROWING PRACTICE
Sit on the floor with your legs apart and place your baby between them with his back to you in Tailor Pose.

Take hold of his arms and open them wide. Move his arms rhythmically back and forth, as if he were rowing a boat, while singing or playing the nursery rhyme.

'Ruben adores singing. Since doing Forward Bend he has become particularly fond of "Row Your Boat" – and he gets to have a good stretch at the same time.'

REBECCA, MOTHER OF RUBEN

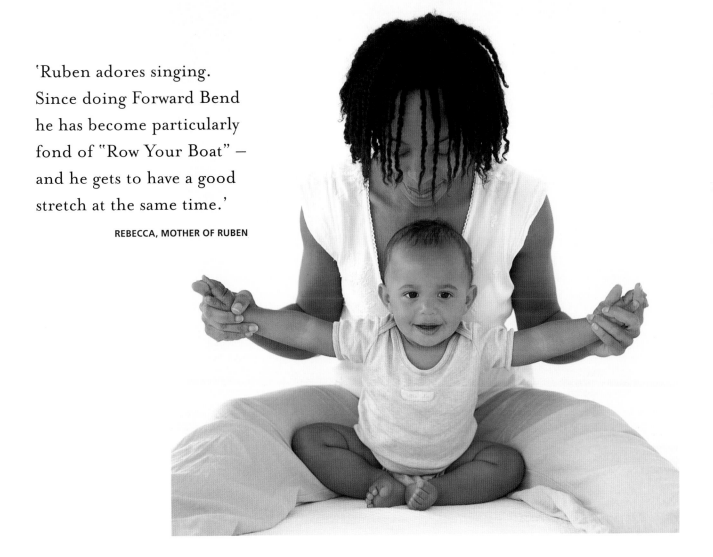

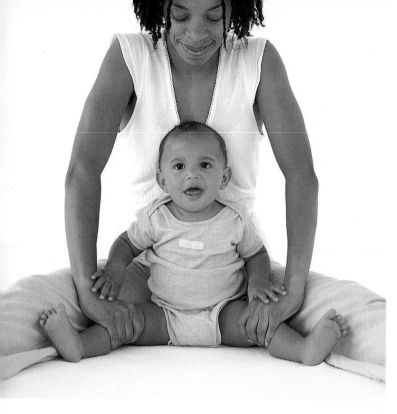

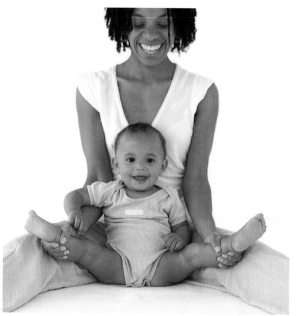

tailor pose to side splits

Opening your baby's legs into side splits can increase his stability
when sitting and enhance the fluidity of his movements.

OPENING UP
Starting from Tailor Pose (see page 56), put your palms
over your baby's knees, take hold of his legs and open
them out into side splits. Fold them in again and repeat
as often as he enjoys. Lightly bounce your baby's knees
up and down to loosen the legs and release tension.
To add to the fun, accompany the action with a nursery
rhyme or a made-up song, or introduce counting.

side splits roll-back

When your baby is relaxed and confident in the movements
he will work well with you and allow you to guide him.

ROLLING BACK
Start from Tailor Pose (see page 56), take hold of your
baby's ankles and roll them back so that his legs come
up off the floor. Again, the rhyme 'Row Your Boat' is a
good accompaniment to the action. Complete as many
roll-backs as your baby is happy to do.

moving side splits

This is a good exercise for stretching the muscles of the calves and thighs, which helps to keep them nice and supple, while at the same time supporting and strengthening the back.

FEELING THE RHYTHM

When your baby starts crawling, the thigh muscles begin to tone and tighten and can restrict flexibility. This activity encourages the muscles to relax while maintaining flexibility. It is a good follow-on from Side Splits Roll-back (see page 64).

Take the opportunity to have a good stretch yourself and synchronize your movements with those of your child. Playing a recording of a favourite nursery rhyme and coordinating the action with the beat and rhythm of the music will help to maintain your child's attention.

KEEPING IN TIME

With your baby in Tailor Pose, place your hands on his ankles. Bend one leg in at a time, then straighten it out again. Keep moving the legs in time with the music. As he comes to enjoy this activity, your baby will be keen to keep repeating it until he has had enough.

'Doing these exercises with Ruben reminds me to take the opportunity to have a good stretch myself.'

REBECCA, MOTHER OF RUBEN

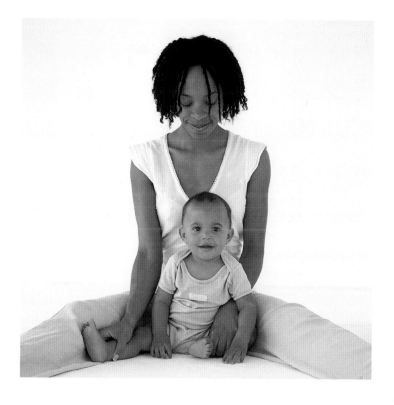

back bend, lift & turn over

Parents tend to be more apprehensive than babies about trying this sequence of movements – which is safe to do from around the early crawling stage, since by then your child will have acquired the right amount of strength and physical development.

CARE AND ATTENTION

These movements are safe for you and your baby to do provided that you always hold the baby's legs around the shins and calves, and not on the ankles. This style of hold eliminates the risk of pulling or over-stretching your child's ankle joints.

THE BENEFITS

A child who is relaxed and willing will get the most from this sequence of movements, which helps to build up strength in the muscles of the hip. You will doubtless notice a 'wow' factor when demonstrating this to friends and family.

As your child learns and you gain confidence, he will grow relaxed in the various positions and become a willing participant, letting you guide and support him through the movements.

Back Bend, Lift & Turn Over follows on naturally from Back Bend and Shoulder Stand, Handstand & Hang, described on pages 58 and 59.

THE SEQUENCE

step 1

Kneel on a rug or cushion or sit in a chair. Follow the steps for Back Bend, as described on page 58. Place your hands just above your baby's ankles.

step 2

Lift your baby up from Back Bend and hold him upside down. Rotate his body to face downwards, so that you can get ready to lie him over your knees.

step 3

Lie your baby down on his front over your lap. He will probably stretch out his arms and place his hands on the floor in front of him.

step 4

Repeat the whole sequence, but this time start with your baby on his front.

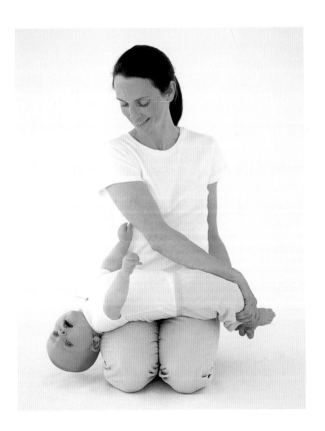

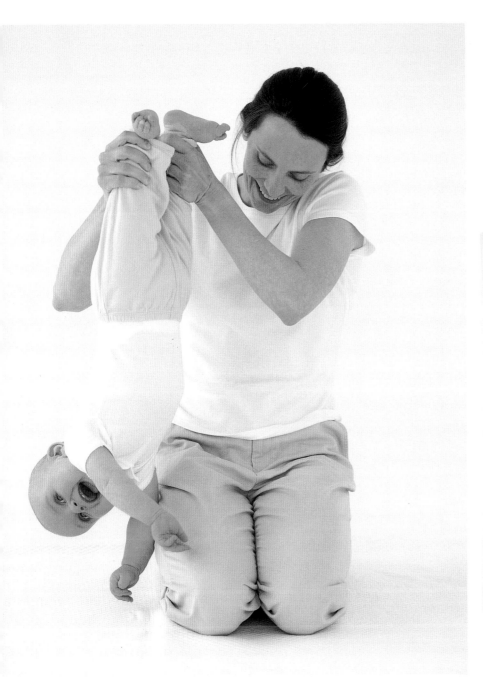

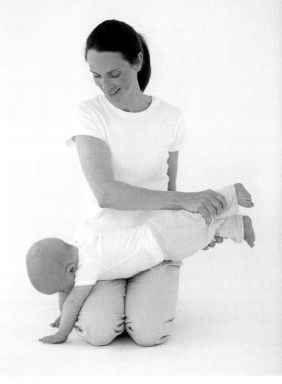

although **parents** may have initial **reservations**, there is
no doubt that **babies love** the sensation of hanging free

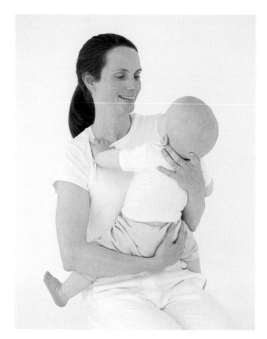

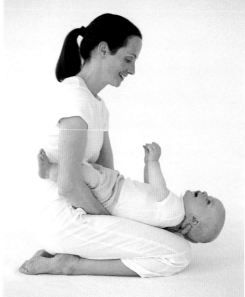

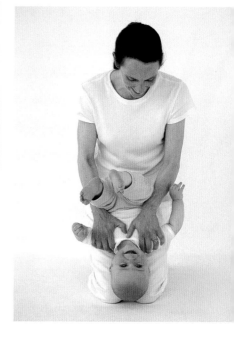

backward tumble

This sequence of movements is a good way to maintain your baby's flexibility and suppleness while encouraging his body to open out, and strengthening his back. It is also great fun for both of you.

ON THE MOVE

Your child may have reached the stage at which he no longer wishes to stay still for massage and is more interested in moving about and exploring the world around him. Doing Backward Tumble and similar movements will help to maintain the healthy bond established between you by the earlier sequences.

A child can start doing Backward Tumble from the age of about seven months – or earlier, depending on his physical development and whether he has grown used to doing Back Bends (see pages 58 and 66–67).

Children of this age enjoy being propelled in motion. As their mobility develops, they learn to roll over and may start to crawl. Gone are the days when you can leave your child and go into the next room and come back to discover him in the same place! Doing yoga movements together will help you to gain trust in your child's ability and potential, which can be a boost to his psychological development.

If your child is not keen to do the sequence, you can encourage him by singing and making sounds that you know he likes. Or try bouncing his body very gently as you lead him into the moves, which will ease tension and help him to relax. When you see that he has had enough, stop, and try again later or on another day.

Your child can do the Backward Tumble sequence while you are in a kneeling position or sitting on a chair or sofa. Choose whichever position helps you to feel

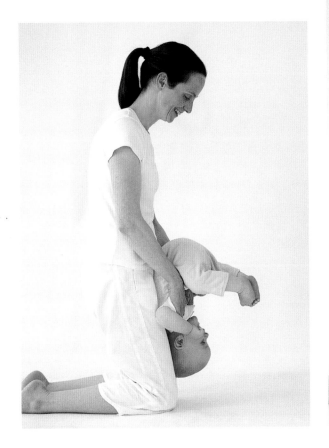

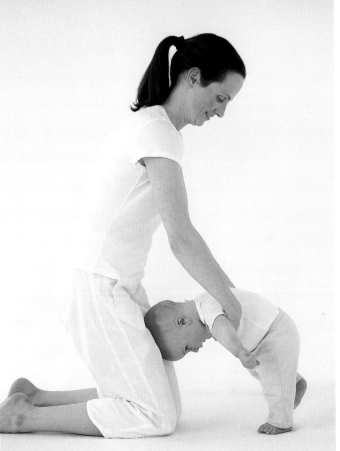

most comfortable and secure. As your child gets bigger, you can try doing the movements while standing.

THE SEQUENCE

step 1

Hug your child to you with his legs wrapped around your waist. Place a supporting hand at the base of his back and the other hand around the back of his head.

step 2

Encourage your child to open up his chest and the front of his body by leaning him right back on your lap in a backward bend. A good way to do this is to lean your body forward over your child, guiding him backwards.

step 3

Place your hands, palms down, on his upper chest and gently take hold of his shoulders. This is a very secure and supporting position for your child. Rise up on your knees to guide his legs up.

step 4

Keeping close to your child to give him reassurance and support, feed his legs up and over through your arms.

step 5

Guide your child's legs back towards the ground, maintaining a good support, until his feet touch the ground. Then bring him up into a standing position.

BACKWARD TUMBLE

standing back bend

This is the first in a series of more vigorous activities that will introduce you and your child to the delights of baby gym. They follow on naturally from the yoga movements covered earlier – but don't try them until you are sure that your child is ready.

THE BENEFITS

Back bends and similar exercises boost coordination, suppleness, flexibility, strength and fluidity of movement.

THE SEQUENCE

step 1

In a standing position, lift up your child and put her legs around your waist. Hug your child to you, stretch out one of your arms and lean her back onto it. When you try this for the first time, you can put a supporting hand under her head and another at the base of her back.

step 2

When you feel confident, let go of your child's head and allow her to hang backwards, then bring her back up into a hug. Repeat as often as she enjoys it.

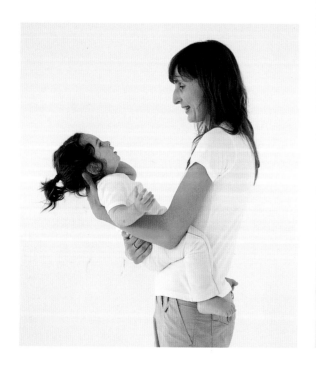

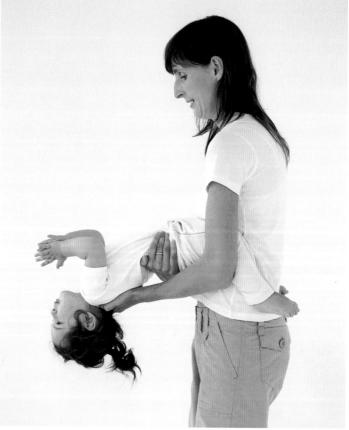

children enjoy an **exhilarating** sense of **freedom**
when they can **hang** and swing **upside down**

swinging back bend

Having mastered the simple back bend, you can then add a swing from side to side to guide your child into a deeper stretch.

LET YOUR CHILD HAVE FUN

With adult support, children can let themselves go and enjoy this wonderful stretch. If you want to try it with your child, make sure that you leave it for at least a couple of hours after a meal – and don't do it unless she is in a good mood and shows a clear willingness to participate.

THE SEQUENCE

step 1

Follow the same sequence as for a Standing Back Bend, as described on page 70.

step 2

Lightly bounce your child up and down with both hands supporting her lower back. This will encourage her into a deeper stretch. Once she is comfortable with this, gently sway her from side to side.

step 3

Bring her back into a hug and then try again as many times as she likes – or as long as the strength in your arms holds out!

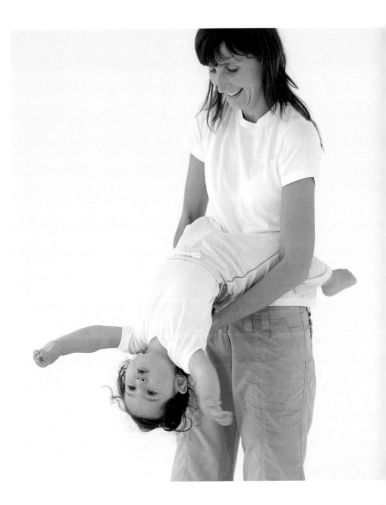

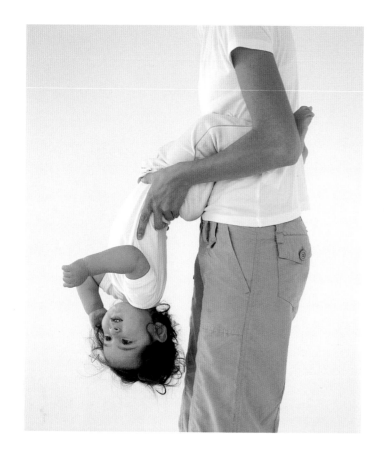

'Ever since she was a small baby, Mazi has always enjoyed hanging upside down. When I held her, she would arch herself backwards, so it's natural for her to do these moves.'

KIRI, MOTHER OF MAZI

back bend to handstand

This sequence gives a wonderful stretch through the back and along the whole body. As your child supports her weight on her hands with your help, she builds up her arm, shoulder and back muscles.

YOUR POSTURE

These movements rely on your holding and supporting your child securely – remember always to pay attention to your own posture and the health of your back. Do not do this exercise with your child if you are suffering from any sort of back problem.

As shown in the left-hand photograph opposite, you can use your thighs for your child to lean on as you guide her towards the ground. Maintaining close bodily contact will give your child confidence and a sense of security. She can then relax into the movement.

DOING IT DIFFERENTLY

As an alternative, you can begin this sequence with your child lying on the floor and lift her into a handstand by holding her legs just above her ankles. Arrange rugs and cushions on the floor around you to ensure a soft landing. This will also help you both to feel more secure.

THE SEQUENCE

step 1

In a standing position, hug your child to you, wrap her legs around your waist and lower her into a Back Bend

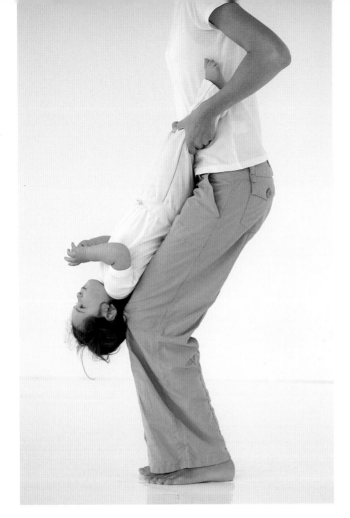
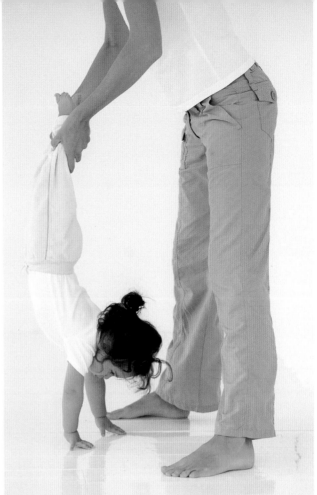

(see page 70). Keeping both your hands on her lower back for support, lean her further back into the stretch.

step 2
As you lean your child back, slide your hands to her hips. This is a very safe hold and you will feel that you have a good grip on her.

step 3
Bend your knees and lower your child down onto your thighs for support. You can then can slide her further

down towards the floor and move your hands up to her knees. She will begin to take her arms back.

step 4
With your hands on her knees, slide them along her legs to just above the ankles. Straighten your knees and hold your child away from you while guiding her hands to the floor in a handstand. From this position, you can bring her body down towards the floor so she is lying on her front. Once she has had a chance to rest, you can, if desired, begin the sequence again.

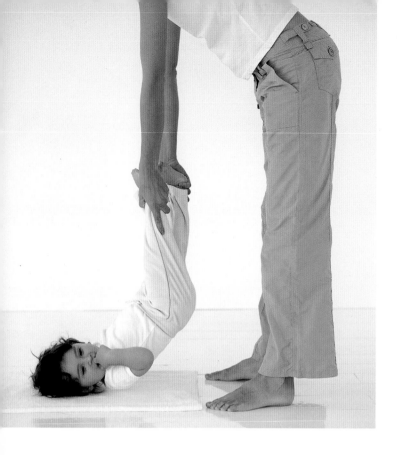

'This exercise is excellent for Mazi since she is able to relax into the shoulder stand. She can also expend a bit of energy and have some fun — and it is strengthening and toning at the same time.'

KIRI, MOTHER OF MAZI

back bend to shoulder stand

This exercise mimics the inversion poses of adult yoga, except that in this case you are assisting your child into the position. Like all such poses, it offers a good counterbalance to long periods of being on the feet.

CONTINUING THE GOOD WORK

As you practise and grow more familiar with Shoulder Stand and the other yoga and gym sequences described in this chapter, you will begin to notice improvements in your child's strength, flexibily, agility, coordination, suppleness, confidence and resilience.

To maintain the good work you have started, it may be worth joining a children's yoga class. When children do not have the opportunity to stretch or benefit from massage, their muscles can tighten, making the joints inflexible. In the long term, this can prove detrimental to good posture in both sitting and standing positions.

WHEN TO TRY SHOULDER STAND

Your child should be at least one year old before you do this exercise with her. By the time she has reached this age, she will have acquired enough language skills and understanding for you to be able to instruct and guide her into the posture, which will make it much easier to win her cooperation.

inversion poses benefit the **circulation** as well as facilitating **release of tension** from the body

THE SEQUENCE

step 1

Start the sequence with a Standing Back Bend (see page 70). From this position, let your child lean right back and lower her until her shoulders are resting on the floor. Support her weight and let her enjoy this stretch. She will let you know when she has had enough and whether she would like to do it again.

step 2

Gently let down your child onto her back on the floor, where you may wish to have a rug and cushions ready for a nice soft landing.

step 3

Repeat the sequence or, as a variation, hold your child just above the ankles and lift her into a Shoulder Stand.

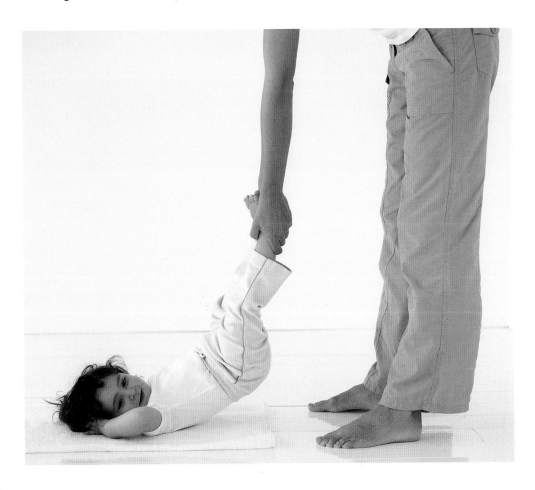

upside-down swing

Tension is released as the spine lengthens during this stretch. It is very important to hold your child's legs just above the ankles.

THE SEQUENCE

step 1

Follow steps for Back Bend to Handstand (see pages 72–73); or ask your child to lie on her back, take hold of her legs just above the ankles, lift and allow her to hang upside down.

step 2

As long as your child is enjoying it, give her a couple of swings from side to side. Then, depending on how happy she is, either repeat the sequence or carry on swinging her gently from side to side.

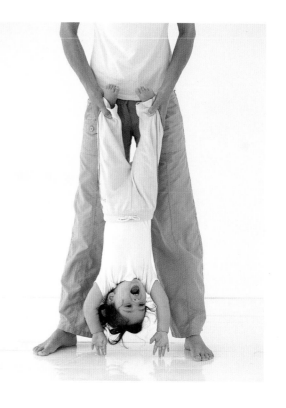

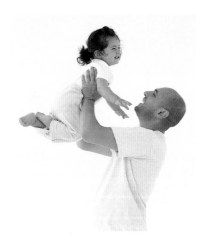

throw and catch

This movement is tremendous fun and most children love it. It will help you to gain confidence in handling your child, as well as improving your child's trust in you.

PURE JOY

It is delightful to watch the expression of a child who enjoys being thrown up into the air and caught. You can try this activity with a baby as young as three to four months, but build up to it gradually, perhaps starting with High Lift (page 62). As long as the child is enjoying it, you can repeat the exercise several times.

THE SEQUENCE

step 1

With your child facing you, hold her under the arms. Start to lift her while counting '1, 2, 3.'

step 2

Throw your child up . . . and catch her!

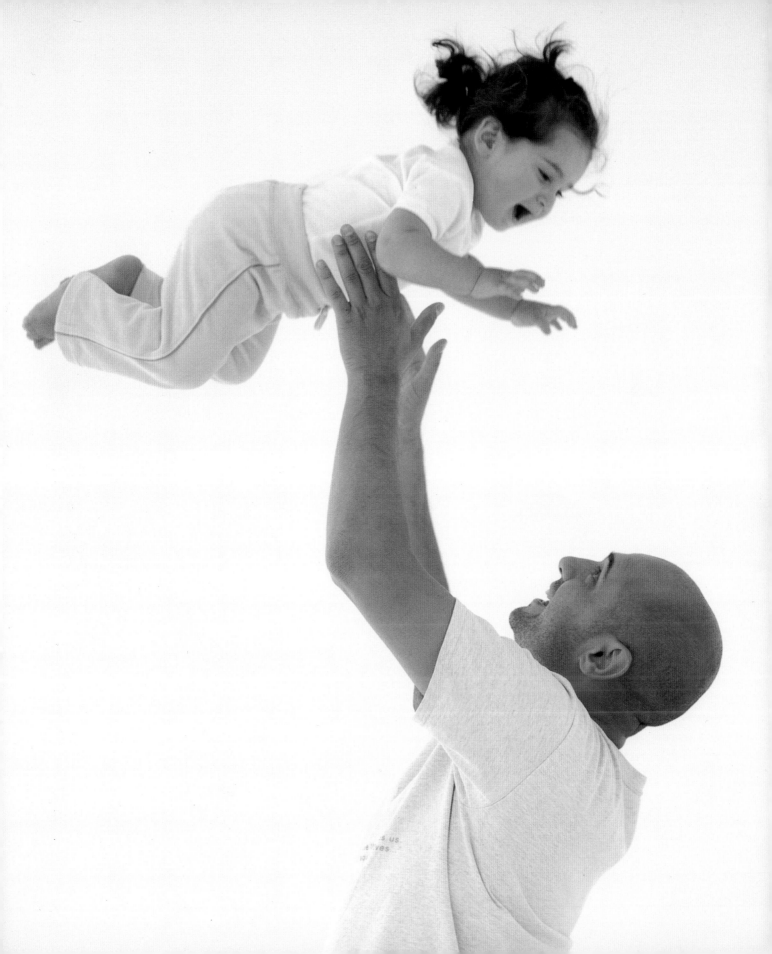

star stretch

Children really love doing Star Stretch, especially when it includes being spun around a few times, but it needs to be performed with special care. To avoid unnecessary pulling or strain on the joints, make sure to hold your child above the ankles and wrists – and not on the joints themselves.

GETTING INTO POSITION

Since you will be picking up and supporting the whole weight of your child, it is important for your own well-being to start this sequence in the right position.

As shown in the photograph below, you should bend your knees and crouch down before taking hold of your child's limbs just above the wrist and ankle.

(Avoid this exercise if you are suffering from any kind of back problem.) Your hand positioning is also crucial for the comfort and safety of your child; take care not to pick him up by the wrist and ankle joints.

Since this exercise is slightly more complicated than the others given in this chapter, it is advisable to try it, at least initially, in a professionally run baby yoga class.

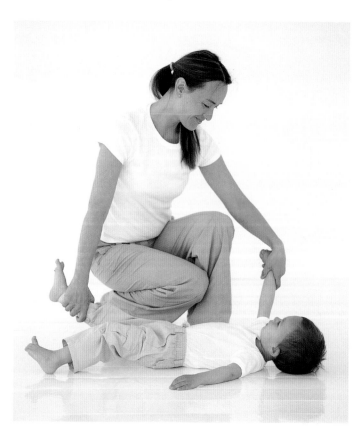

THE SEQUENCE

step 1

With your child lying on his back on the floor and you crouching down on his right side facing him, take hold of his right arm and his right leg.

step 2

Lift up your child, then lie him gently back down on the floor.

step 3

Lift him up again and swing him gently from side to side three or four times, or until he has had enough.

step 4

Swing him round in a circle, then lie him gently back down on the floor.

step 5

To even out the stretch, repeat on the other side.

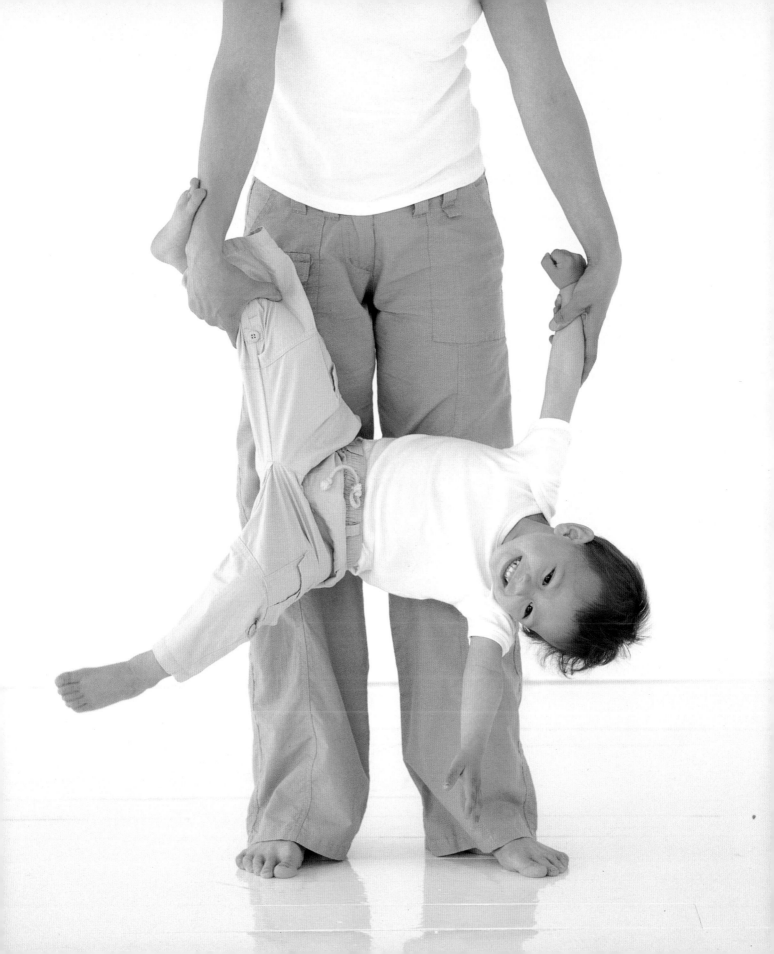

Baby yoga and gym are hugely enjoyable activities in themselves – but there are many ways in which you can enhance your baby's relaxation and exercise sessions so that both of you have even more fun.

I One of the most productive ways to engage with your baby and to build up a relationship of mutual trust is through speech. If you talk to your baby about the movements you are doing together – describing and commenting on them – it will encourage the baby to respond by chatting back. Soon your baby will take the lead when it comes to deciding which exercises to do!

TEN WAYS TO...*have more fun*

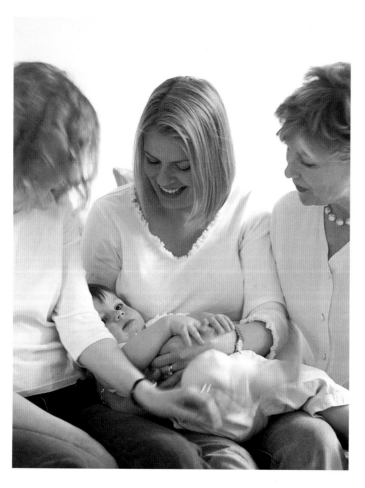

2 Play music to accompany your yoga and gym movements. Children love music, and anything from Mozart to their favourite television show themes can help to set the right mood. Music provides a background rhythm and tempo against which to do the exercises – especially good when you are repeating the movements.

3 Singing is an excellent way to encourage your child to learn nursery rhymes and lyrics and acquire a sense of rhythm. 'Row Your Boat' goes well with Forward Bend (page 63) and 'Head, Shoulders, Knees and Toes' makes a good accompaniment to Side Splits (page 64). Your child will learn to associate some of the yoga and gym movements with particular songs – and remember what to do next time the sounds are heard.

4 Invite other members of the family to become involved with the yoga and gym activities you are planning. This is a wonderful way to encourage family members to interact physically with your child, and will reinforce their confidence in handling the new arrival. From grandmother and grandfather to aunts, uncles and siblings, everyone is sure to have a great time.

5 As a baby develops greater mobility, a father's confidence in handling the baby usually increases. Seize the chance offered by baby yoga and gym sessions to encourage good-quality 'dad time'. Allow your partner to participate in as many activities as possible that involve physical interaction with the baby.

6 Laugh with your baby. Laughing and making eye contact while doing yoga and gym are wonderfully nurturing ways of communicating. Laughter is also good for the soul and helps to boost the immune system.

7 Play games. Be creative and make up games linked to your baby yoga and gym exercises. Drawing on the Tailor Pose Swing (page 57), you could try 'Flying Aeroplanes', or with Throw and Catch (pages 76–77) you could play 'Zooming Rockets'.

8 Use a mirror. Children thoroughly enjoy seeing their reflection in the mirror while doing an Upside-down Swing (page 76) or a Star Stretch (pages 78–79). You can also incorporate a mirror in games such as 'Now you see me, now you don't'.

9 Take advantage of the great outdoors. When the weather is fine and warm enough for you and your baby to be outside, seize the opportunity to spread out and make use of the space in your garden or local park for your baby yoga and gym exercises. If you visit the park on a regular basis, your child might even make some new friends.

IO Organize get-togethers with other children and their parents. Children generally enjoy activities that involve other people, which makes it more enjoyable for all concerned. Guide your child to use this time for learning, having fun and socializing.

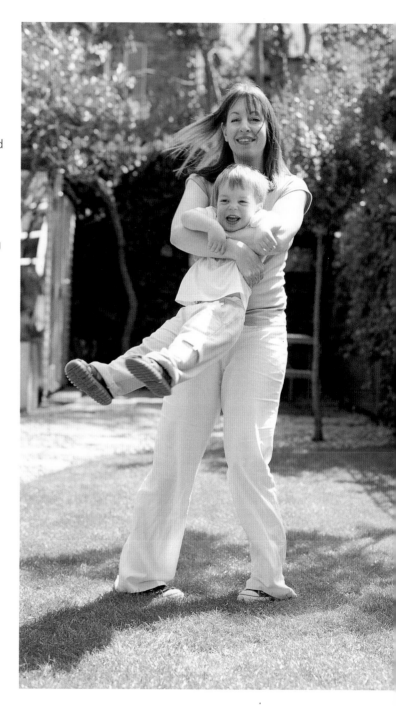

your questions answered

It is a pleasure to observe a child who appears to be completely comfortable with his or her body, and who is able to express this sense of ease through agility and freedom of movement.

WHAT ARE THE BENEFITS TO MY CHILD OF DOING YOGA AND GYM?

These activities encourage a healthy posture and spine. A position such as Tailor Pose (see page 56) encourages the development of a good postural habit that will stand your child in good stead when older. Increased strength and agility in the body can help to prepare children for other sports and may encourage you to take them to a children's yoga class.

ARE THERE TIMES WHEN SHOULD I AVOID DOING YOGA OR GYM WITH MY CHILD?

A child who is ill will not like doing yoga or gym. When children have just eaten, they should be allowed some time to digest before taking part in physical activity. A child who is too tired or over-stimulated may not enjoy yoga or gym, and you won't have a good time either!

HOW OFTEN SHOULD WE DO BABY YOGA AND GYM?

You could have a session once a day – or when you feel like it. Many parents like to incorporate it into the daily routine, which can help to structure the day's activities.

WHEN IS THE BEST TIME TO DO THE MOVEMENTS?

Any time. A good time to try is when your child is alert and happy. Observe your child and be guided by him or her. You will then get the best from the experience.

CAN THE POSTURES DO ANY HARM TO MY BABY?

As long as they are performed correctly, the postures and movements described in this chapter will not do any harm to your baby. When trying the movements for the first time, use a mat or cushions for extra safety. If you are at all unsure about the correct hold or position to adopt, join a baby yoga class and seek expert advice.

CAN BABY YOGA OR GYM CAUSE ME HARM?

As long as you pay attention to your posture and the way in which you use your body, baby yoga and gym will not harm you. It is important to adopt the correct stance and hold, and to use the support of cushions, mats and chairs when doing some of the holds and swings. In Tailor Pose Swing (page 57), what feels best is having your baby perfectly balanced in the posture, so that there is no strain in your shoulders or back.

baby yoga and baby gym involve your child in **physical activities** that can have a crucial and long-lasting influence on **health, happiness and well-being**

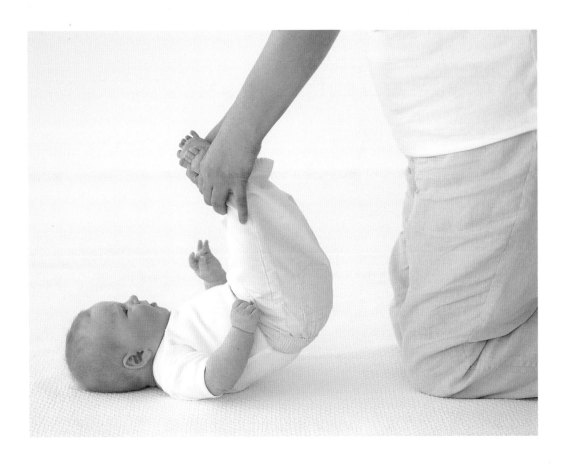

WHAT SHOULD I DO IF MY BABY CRIES WHILE DOING YOGA OR GYM?

If your baby cries while you are doing the movements, stop and settle him or her. It may be that the baby is hungry, tired, agitated or simply does not wish to do any more. Respond to your child's wishes. You can try the movements again when the baby is settled or leave it for another time. Again, be guided by your child.

WHAT IF MY BABY DOESN'T LIKE DOING SOME OF THE POSTURES OR MOVEMENTS?

There may be times when your child is not happy to do some of the movements or postures, particularly the first time you try them. With practice, you and your child will get to know the movements and enjoy them more, especially when you both gain confidence. If it is clear that your child does not want to do a particular

movement, that is OK. Move on to another movement – and try the original one again on another occasion.

SHOULD I AVOID ANY PARTICULAR MOVEMENTS?

No, unless your child has a physical condition such as a dislocating hip. If necessary, seek professional advice. Also, be guided by the stage your child has reached in terms of development. The strength and control that children have over their bodies will determine their ability to do some of the movements and not others.

UNTIL WHAT AGE CAN A CHILD DO YOGA AND GYM?

There is no particular cut-off point, so be guided by your child. You may find that a child becomes too big or heavy to do some of the movements, such as Tailor Pose Swing. To nurture your child further, you could try to find a suitable children's yoga class.

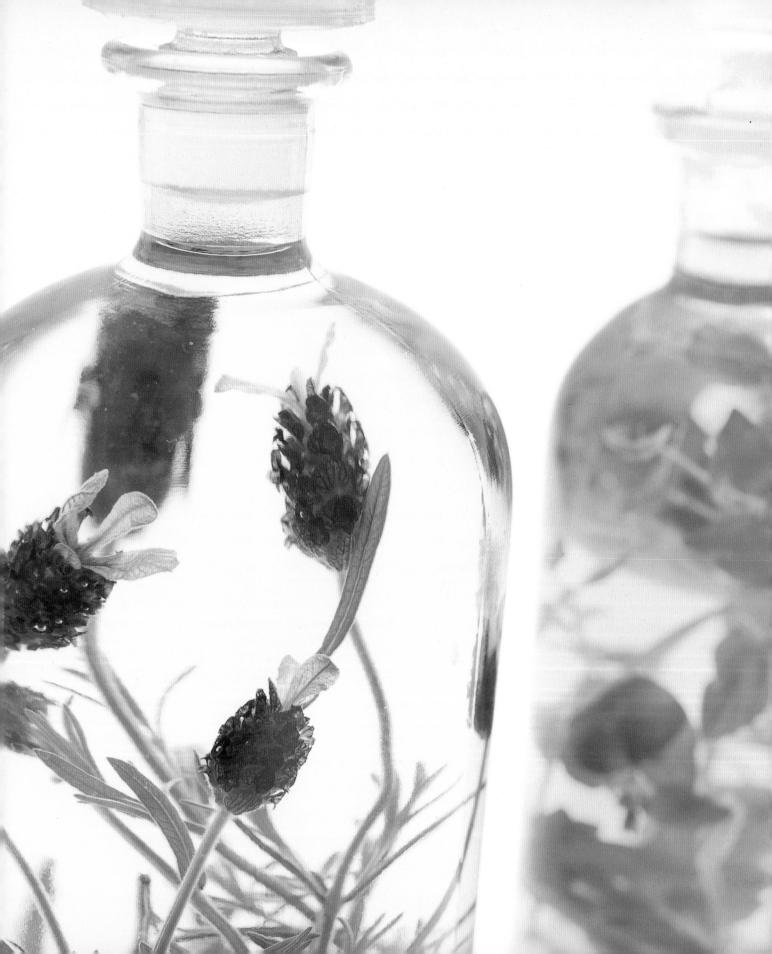

baby aromatherapy

Aromatherapy is the gentle art of using pure essential oils in therapeutic ways. Babies can enjoy its benefits by means of massage or diffusion – or by having a few drops of diluted essential oil added to their baths. This chapter explains how to create blissful moments for you and your baby by making the most of nature's fragrant gifts.

sharing natural scents

A baby's sense of smell is as acute as that of a pregnant or breastfeeding woman, and sharing the pleasure of natural scents that simply kiss the air is a lovely way to bond with your baby. Aromatherapy allows you both to benefit from this fragrant link in a way that is both gentle and effective.

AROMATIC MAGIC

As an aromatherapist and a mother of two, I used aromatherapy throughout my pregnancies and on both my babies. Those 'babies' are now aged 19 and 14, and all three of us continue to use essential oils on a daily basis. I don't know what I would have done when they were tiny without my basic kit of essential oils to deal with niggly baby troubles from nappy rash to croup. At the first sign of a major problem, I consulted my doctor or pharmacist, but aromatherapy helped me to keep at bay many of the little problems that can grow more serious if allowed to get out of control.

AN ANCIENT ART

Traces of essential oils have been discovered in ancient Egyptian burial chambers, and depictions of diffusion are clearly apparent in murals dating back to the Stone Age. The tradition of burning herbs and spices for their fragrant and sometimes hypnotic effects gave rise to the word perfume, which derives from the phrase *per fume*, meaning 'through fire'.

More recent associations draw on memories of our mothers or grandmothers using nature's pharmacy as a source of basic aids in the home: for example, lavender to scent clothes, cedar wood to deter moths, cloves to alleviate toothache, lemon to disinfect.

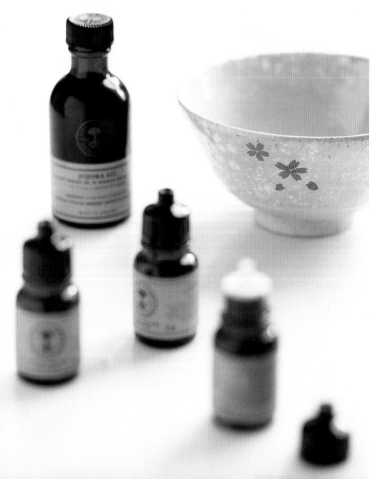

WHAT IS DISTINCTIVE ABOUT ESSENTIAL OILS?

Most baby products are made from mineral oils that form a barrier between the skin and the air. Unless the skin is absolutely dry and clean, this can cause problems such as cradle cap and nappy rash.

By contrast, dilute blends of essential oils are subtly absorbed into the deeper layers of the skin, letting the skin breathe while being conditioned and nourished. At the same time, their therapeutic properties promote well-being and can ease minor ailments. When essential oils are inhaled, they affect the limbic area of the brain, which is associated with mood and emotion; this means that the sense of smell can be used as a powerful tool when trying to calm a baby.

AROMATHERAPY BASICS

Essential oils should always be diluted with a vegetable carrier oil before being used on a baby's skin; as little as 2 drops of essential oil can be added to a dessertspoon of carrier oil. Essential oils do not dissolve well in water, so, before using them in a baby's bath, dilute by adding 2 drops of essential oil to a teaspoon of full-fat milk.

Any blends that you want to keep should be stored in brown, blue or, less commonly, green glass bottles since essential oils are light-sensitive and will deteriorate if exposed to bright light. Lids should be kept closed when not in use – if they are left off for long periods, blends will become rancid and less effective. Blends can be kept for approximately six months, but it is better to make small amounts and use them within a few weeks. Essential oils, carrier oils and glass bottles are usually available from chemists and health-food shops.

Alternatively, you can buy ready-made aromatherapy blends for babies. These tend to last longer than home-made ones because they often include Vitamin E, which is a natural preservative as well as being good for the skin. Choose a brand that offers clear instructions and ingredients listings along with a telephone advice line.

FOLLOW YOUR INSTINCT

The essential oils described in this chapter can be used from birth, with the exception of lime, which has a more powerful aroma than the others and would be better saved until your baby is a few months old and has experienced a wider array of naturally occurring scents. Lime also has slightly astringent properties that are not needed in the first few months of a baby's life.

Once diluted, lime would do no harm to a newborn baby, but fragrances that are too strong can agitate and cause irritability. Such as reaction goes against the natural thrust of baby aromatherapy – which should dovetail naturally into your infant's routine without causing any upset.

The dilutions given on the following pages are so gentle that they present no danger, but, if you are at all unsure, wait until you feel the time is right. A parent's instinct is paramount.

GETTING STARTED

If you are new to baby aromatherapy, here are a few words of advice.

□ Ensure that you keep essential oils out of the reach of children, with lids or tops on bottles, out of direct sunlight and in a relatively cool environment.

□ Less is more. Never use more for greater effect. It doesn't work like that.

□ Never take or give essential oils internally.

□ Have fun with your essential oils – but respect them.

knowledge of the benefits of **myrtle, chamomile and dill** has been handed down through the ages

'On Glenda's advice, I used essential oils on my children from the very start with utter confidence. I loved it so much that I went on to train as an aromatherapist!'

GEORGINA, MOTHER OF IRVIN AND BARNIE

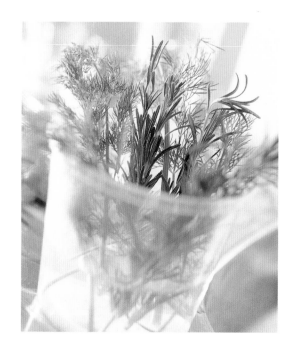

which oils are best for babies?

Here are some of the best essential oils to use in baby aromatherapy. They need to be carefully diluted for massage and bath. Once you have learned the principles of diluting essential oils, you can feel confident in creating your own combinations.

CARRIER OILS

To make essential oils safe for application to the skin or for use in the bath, they must be diluted in carrier oils. In baby aromatherapy, vegetable oils should be used for this purpose rather than baby oil, which is a mineral oil and will stay on the surface of the skin, preventing the essential oils from working properly. Light, odourless carrier oils include sunflower, grapeseed and almond (though some people prefer to avoid almond and other nut-based oils because of the risk of promoting allergy).

Jojoba, another carrier oil, has a rich consistency similar to liquid wax. It can be used on its own to treat really troublesome skin. More commonly, it is mixed with sunflower, grapeseed or almond in a 10 per cent proportion, to make a slightly richer carrier oil.

BENZOIN

Benzoin, derived from benjamin, makes an oil that is thick and viscous, with a fragrance that recalls vanilla – sweet and medicinal, but at the same time very subtle. It is perfect for soothing skins that are itchy or sore.

CHAMOMILE

Along with lavender, chamomile is one of the essential oils most frequently used in baby aromatherapy. It is very soothing and contains azulene, a natural painkiller.

DILL

The light aniseed-like fragrance of dill is calming and particularly useful for resolving digestive problems. Dill is one of the main active ingredients of gripe water.

LAVENDER

Regarded as a 'cleansing' oil, lavender is antibacterial and antiviral, making it efficient at warding off germs. (The word lavender comes from the Latin for 'to wash'.) Although widely thought to have a relaxing effect, lavender is actually a synergistic oil. This means that it adapts to the situation it is in. For example, if you use lavender with chamomile, its effect is relaxing; if you use it with lime, its effect is more uplifting.

LIME

Lime is a wonderful oil to use in summer when the weather is hot because its effect is cooling and refreshing. It has a 'playful' fragrance reminiscent of sweets. Wait until your baby is at least two or three months old before using lime.

MANDARIN

Mandarin is known in France as the children's oil. It is the most gentle of all essential oils and has a 'happy', euphoric effect without being stimulating. You could bathe your baby in the evening in a mandarin bath without fear of making him or her too alert for sleep.

MYRTLE

Traditionally included in bridal bouquets to bring luck, myrtle is from the same family as eucalyptus, but, unlike eucalyptus, which is stimulating, myrtle is calming and soothing while still working as a gentle decongestant.

NEROLI

Known for its ability to calm nerves, neroli is another traditional constituent of bridal bouquets. Although it is not commonly used in baby aromatherapy, its gentle action is perfect for soothing restless babies. Neroli can reassure a mother about her femininity while allowing her to share a calming experience with her baby.

ROSE

Similar to neroli in that it is rather more sophisticated than most of the oils that are commonly used in baby aromatherapy, rose is a lovely oil to use when a little bit of luxury is called for.

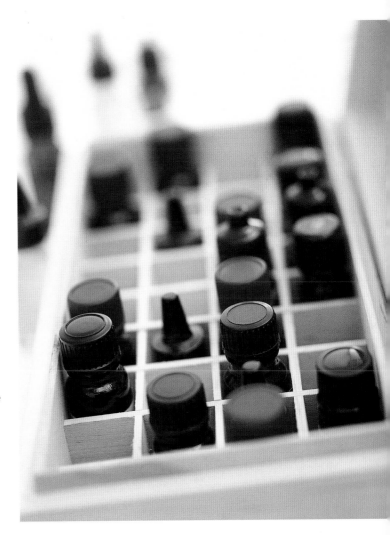

diffusing essential oils

Diffusion of essential oils creates a gently fragrant atmosphere while allowing the oils to release their therapeutic vapours. The simple combinations of oils suggested here can change the mood of a room in an instant. Diffusion can also cleanse the atmosphere and help to combat airborne microbes.

ELECTRIC VAPORIZERS

The most effective way to diffuse essential oils is by means of an electric vaporizer. Vaporizers are safe to use and keep the oils at a low temperature, allowing their fragrance to be released gradually into the ambient environment. If you do not possess an electric vaporizer, you can simply add a few drops of essential oil to a bowl of warm water and leave it to stand, or put a few drops of oil onto a handkerchief or tissue and place it on a central-heating radiator.

You can leave an electric vaporizer on for the whole night. They are cheap to run and, since they keep the oils at a constantly low temperature, the relaxing and soothing atmosphere will persist for many hours.

If you are in a large room, or if the essential oils are not in close proximity to your baby, the quantities given below can be doubled.

BEDTIME

To create a relaxed atmosphere in your baby's room that will be conducive to sound sleep.

Chamomile	1 drop
Lavender	2 drops

EASING SNUFFLES

For when your baby has a blocked-up nose and needs help to fight off germs.

Lavender	1 drop
Myrtle	2 drops

PAMPERING

For when your partner gets home and you want to feel grown up and sophisticated after a long hard day.

Neroli	1 drop
Rose	2 drops

PLAYTIME FUN

For when you have other new mothers round to visit and would like everyone to be in a really good mood.

Lime	1 drop
Mandarin	2 drops

SOOTHING

For when you or your partner feel a particular need to share a cosy atmosphere with your baby.

Benzoin	2 drops
Rose	1 drop

response to a familiar **fragrance** can lull your baby into a **receptive** mood for **sleep or play**

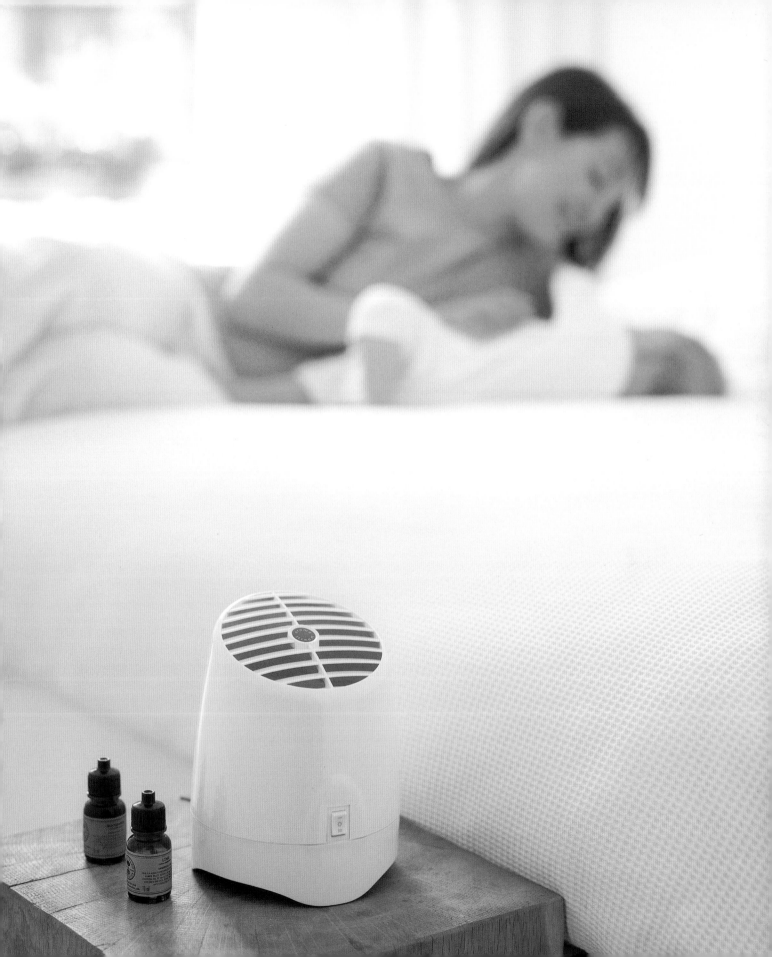

blissful bathtime

Half fill your baby's bath with warm water and choose one of the following blends to add to the water. Agitate the water to ensure even distribution of the oils before putting your baby into the bath.

DISSOLVING THE OILS

Essential oils do not dissolve well in water, especially in the lukewarm water usually used for bathing babies. You can resolve this problem by adding the essential oils to a teaspoon of full-fat milk before putting them in the bath. Just two drops of essential oil in milk is sufficient for a baby's bath.

MASSAGE BLENDS

To create aromatherapy massage blends, use any of the recipes given in this section and replace the teaspoon of milk with a dessertspoon of a carrier oil such as grapeseed, sunflower or almond.

ANY TIME

For babies who just love having an enjoyable splash around, add the following essential oils to one teaspoon of milk:

Lime	1 drop
Mandarin	1 drop

GRUMPY TIME

For babies who are disgruntled for no apparent reason, add the following essential oils to one teaspoon of milk:

Chamomile	1 drop
Dill	1 drop

MORNING TIME

For babies who like to have a bath in the morning to freshen up – and maybe even to go back to sleep afterwards! – add the following essential oils to one teaspoon of milk:

Mandarin	1 drop
Neroli	1 drop

SLEEPY HEAD

To give your baby a lovely all-over relaxed feeling and to encourage blissful sleep, add the following essential oils to one teaspoon of milk:

Chamomile	1 drop
Lavender	1 drop

DOUBLE DELIGHT

The blends described opposite are effective either when used in the bath (when the oils are diluted in milk) or for a massage (when a carrier oil is used), but you can intensify the pleasure by making a massage blend to match your baby's aromatherapy bath. The association of beautiful fragrances with a pleasurable experience will make bathtime sheer bliss for both of you.

After patting your baby dry with a warm fluffy towel, spend a little time massaging her with an aromatherapy blend made from the same essential oils that you used in her bath. Massage your baby's feet, hands, back or abdominal area. There is no need to massage her all over – give attention to those parts of the body that may benefit from extra conditioning or the areas where your baby enjoys being massaged most.

Remember that massage has a stimulating effect, so don't give your baby a massage just before she is due to go to sleep. For in-depth information about baby massage, see pages 22–51.

'Daniel always seemed to have a grumpy time in the late afternoon. I found that giving him a bath around that time with a drop or two of chamomile and dill had an amazingly relaxing effect.'

CAROLINE, MOTHER OF DANIEL

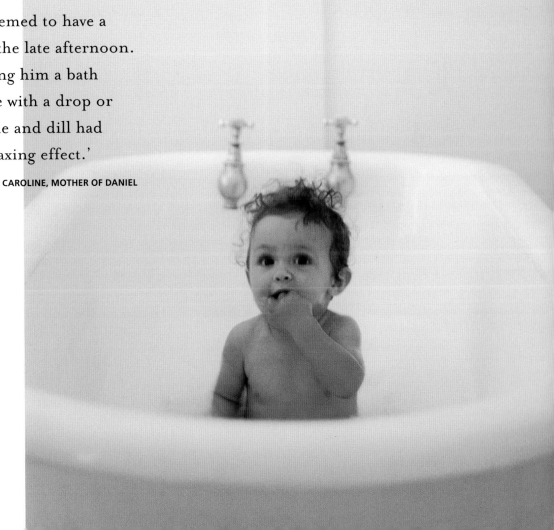

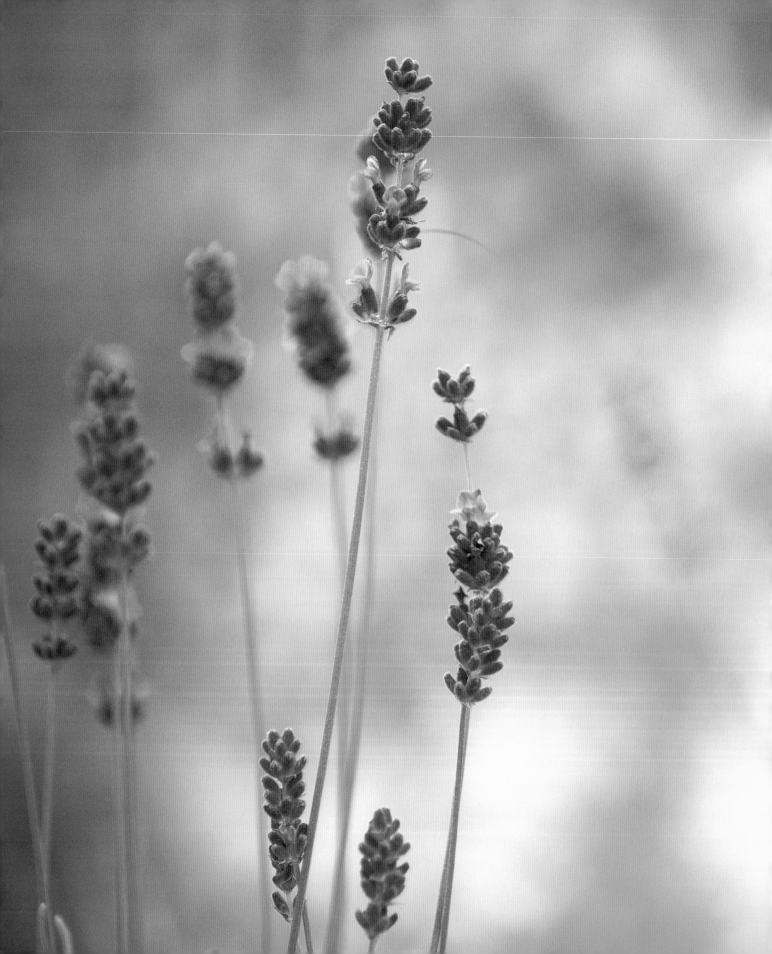

scenting, healing & soothing

Apart from their effects on mood and atmosphere, aromatherapy blends have a part to play in many different aspects of everyday life affecting you and your baby. Here are some alternative ideas.

CLOTHES RINSE

If you wash your baby's clothes by hand, add 1 or 2 drops of essential oil to the final rinse to leave a gentle lingering fragrance. Try one of the following mixtures.

Lavender	1 drop
Mandarin	1 drop
or	
Lavender	1 drop
Rose	1 drop

BANISHING HEADLICE

Many school-age children have headlice, or nits, so a baby who comes into contact with older children is susceptible to catching them. This is hard to deal with if your baby has a lot of hair. Anti-headlice chemicals are not suitable for use on a tiny baby. But essential oils are an excellent deterrent to lice, and when correctly diluted are far gentler than commercial preparations. Make up the blend below and rub it gently into your baby's scalp after bathing. There is no need to wash it out. You can keep the remainder in an airtight bottle and use it again a couple of days later. (Some people prefer to avoid almond and other nut-based oils in case they provoke sensitization and later allergy.)

As well as preventing lice, this blend can be used in conjunction with a nit comb to eliminate them. It is also suitable for older children; if the infestation is heavy, use double the quantity of oils for children over two.

Almond or grapeseed	1 dessertspoon
Chamomile or myrtle	1 drop
Lavender	1 drop

CRADLE CAP

Make up a small bottle of the following blend and apply a little to your baby's scalp each day to counteract the yellow, scaly patches of skin known as cradle cap. There is no need to wash it out.

Jojoba	1 dessertspoon
Benzoin	1 drop
Lavender	1 drop

CONSTIPATION

Babies may become constipated when they begin to have milk from a bottle or take their first solid foods. Use the following blend to massage the baby's abdominal area. It may also benefit babies with colic. (See caution about nut-based oils in left-hand column under Banishing Headlice.)

Massage gently with a circular motion and in a clockwise direction, then once or twice in a reverse direction, then clockwise a few more times.

Almond or grapeseed	1 dessertspoon
Dill	1 drop
Mandarin	1 drop

NAPPY RASH

Application of jojoba is one of the most effective ways both to prevent and to treat nappy rash. It moisturizes and nourishes babies' delicate skin while still allowing it to breath. The inclusion of essential oils enhances the actions of the jojoba.

Jojoba	1 dessertspoon
Chamomile or lavender	1 drop

remedies for common baby ailments

This chart shows you at a glance which essential oils are useful for treating common baby ailments – and indicates which methods of application are appropriate in each case. Don't forget that essential oils must always be diluted before coming into contact with a baby's skin. Full instructions for dilution are given on pages 90 and 92.

ailment	essential oils to use	methods of application
allergies	chamomile	bath, diffusion, massage
anxiety	benzoin, chamomile, lavender, mandarin, neroli, rose	bath, diffusion, massage
eczema	benzoin, chamomile, lavender	bath, massage
colic	chamomile, dill, mandarin	massage
constipation	chamomile, dill, mandarin	massage
congestion	myrtle	diffusion, massage
cradle cap	benzoin, chamomile, lavender	massage
croup	benzoin, myrtle	bath, diffusion, massage

ailment	essential oils to use	methods of application
dermatitis	benzoin, chamomile, lavender, rose	bath massage
diarrhoea	chamomile, dill, lavender	bath, diffusion
eczema	benzoin, chamomile, lavender, neroli, rose	bath, massage
feeding problems	chamomile, dill, lavender	diffusion, massage
grumpiness	benzoin, chamomile, lavender, mandarin, neroli, rose	bath, diffusion, massage
headlice/nits	chamomile, lavender, myrtle, rose	bath, massage
heat rash	chamomile, lavender	cool bath
nappy rash	benzoin, chamomile, lavender	bath, massage
sickness	chamomile, dill, lavender, mandarin	bath, diffusion, massage
sleeplessness	chamomile, lavender	bath, diffusion, massage
stings & bites	lavender	bath, massage; if a bite or sting is very bad, a tiny drop of lavender may be used neat in this instance
tiredness	mandarin	bath, diffusion

your questions answered

The concept of aromatherapy for babies tends to throw up many questions. Many of these have been covered earlier in the chapter, but here are the answers to a few more that often arise.

WHEN IS A BABY OLD ENOUGH TO BE GIVEN AROMATHERAPY?

Newborn babies have few requirements apart from love, warmth and nourishment. However, new parents are encouraged to use commercial skin products on their babies almost from birth. Aromatherapy used in the ways described in this chapter is far gentler than anything available commercially – so, with that in mind, baby aromatherapy can be administered from soon after birth, as long as it is done with care.

ARE SOME TIMES OF THE DAY BETTER THAN OTHERS?

The time of day when you prefer to use aromatherapy depends entirely on you and your baby. Never attempt to force the situation. If your baby does not take to aromatherapy initially, leave it for a while and try again another time.

It is important that both you and your baby enjoy the experience, so rely on your instincts and you will most probably find that your baby will follow suit. You may find that both of you will develop specific fragrance preferences at certain times of the day.

SHOULD I COMBINE AROMATHERAPY WITH BABY MASSAGE OR BABY YOGA?

It is an excellent idea to combine aromatherapy with baby massage or yoga. Using a baby aromatherapy blend in baby massage can enhance the benefits of the massage. Likewise, diffusing essential oils during a session of baby yoga or gym can enhance the effectiveness of the movements.

IS THERE ANY DANGER OF AN ALLERGIC REACTION TO AN ESSENTIAL OIL?

As long as you follow the instructions outlined in this chapter, there is no more likelihood of your baby developing an allergic reaction to an essential oil than to any other baby product. Avoid nut-based oils if you are concerned about their possible link with allergy.

IF I USE AROMATHERAPY WHILE BREASTFEEDING, CAN IT HAVE AN ADVERSE EFFECT ON THE FEEDING?

Mothers should exercise care about their choice of essential oils while breastfeeding since some oils have contraindications for use on or in the vicinity of babies. None of the essential oils included in this chapter should present any problem – and this applies to quite a few others – but it is worth taking an aromatherapist's advice before using any that are not mentioned here.

CAN AROMATHERAPY SOLVE FEEDING PROBLEMS?

When feeding difficulties stem from anxiety on the part of either the mother or the baby, aromatherapy can be very helpful in alleviating the problem. (There may, of course, be some other, more complicated reason why feeding is not going well, in which case you should consult your doctor.)

The most effective approach would be to create a calm atmosphere by diffusing a blend of oils in your baby's bedroom. Suitable blends would include the Soothing blend described on page 90 and the Grumpy Time blend described on page 92; the latter contains dill, which can stimulate appetite.

WHAT WILL HAPPEN IF I USE AN ESSENTIAL OIL NOT RECOMMENDED FOR BABIES?

Prolonged use of an inappropriate oil could make a baby very uncomfortable and potentially quite ill. An isolated mistake is not a cause for alarm, however.

WHAT HAPPENS IF I USE A BLEND THAT IS TOO STRONG ON MY BABY?

Depending on the strength of the blend, it will have a progressively more irritant effect and may lead to sickness or diarrhoea.

If you realize that you have exposed your baby to a blend that is too strong, bathe the baby immediately in a cool bath to remove any excess and let him or her drink plenty of water or milk. As long as you do not continue to use a blend that is too strong, there is no need to worry.

WHAT SHOULD I DO IF NEAT ESSENTIAL OIL COMES INTO CONTACT WITH MY BABY'S SKIN?

Wash off the oil with plenty of cool water. In normal circumstances, essential oils should never be used neat on a baby – but a baby stung by a wasp or suffering a small burn may benefit from one drop of neat lavender essential oil applied to the affected area.

FOR HOW LONG CAN I STORE A HOME-MADE BLEND?

As long as you store any blend you have made up in a bottle with the lid or top on, and keep it in a cool environment and well away from direct sunlight, it will last for several months.

IS AROMATHERAPY USEFUL FOR OLDER BABIES AND TODDLERS?

Older babies, and toddlers in particular, are curious about scent and tend to be receptive to aromatherapy, so it can be very effective in helping to calm toddler tantrums or when used as basic first aid. Children will be fascinated by the connection between situations and fragrances, and will probably continue to enjoy aromatherapy when they are much older. (However, you must take great care to keep essential oils out of reach of children since their curiosity may make the oils a temptation too hard to resist.)

You will need to expand your knowledge of essential oils as your children grow up since there are many different varieties that you can incorporate as they get older. The uses described here are just the beginning!

WHAT SHOULD I DO IF A TODDLER DRINKS ESSENTIAL OIL?

Get the toddler to drink plenty of milk and contact your doctor stating exactly what has been consumed.

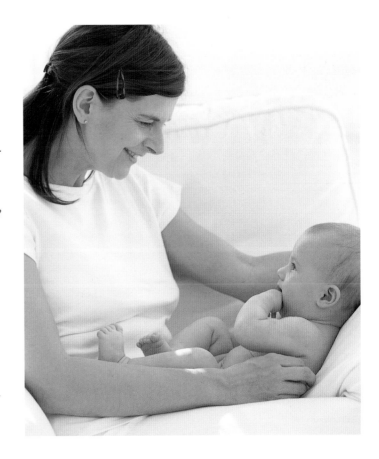

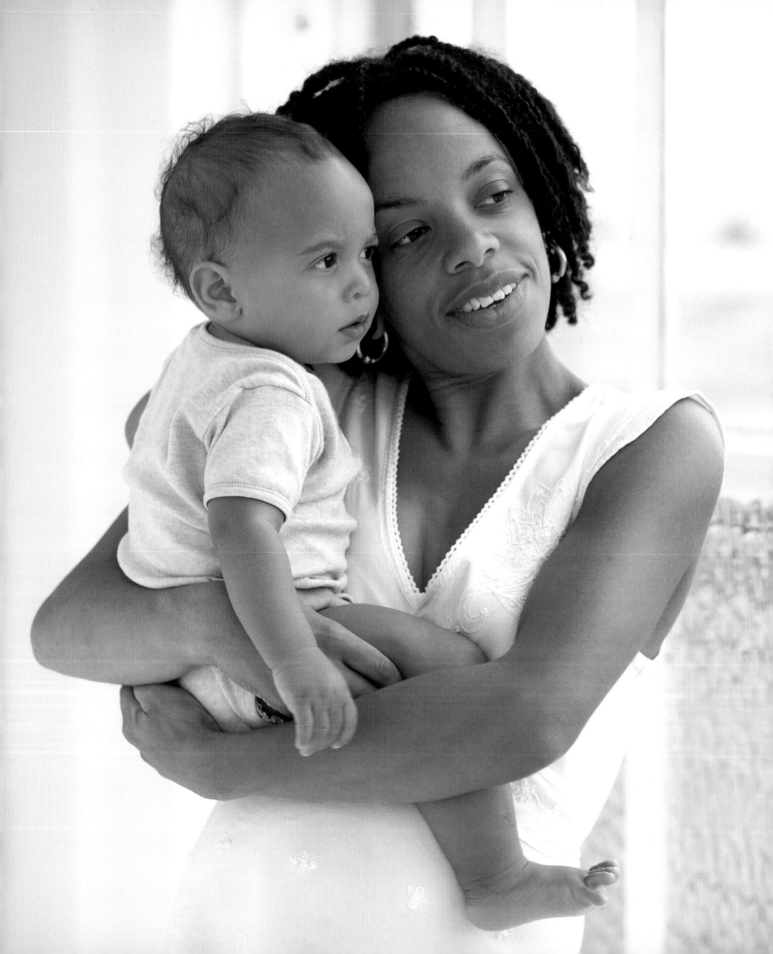

other gentle therapies

Most babies love being in water, and bathing,
perhaps combined with aromatherapy, can soothe
when necessary, as well as giving opportunities
for play. Reflexology, homeopathy, Bach Flower
Remedies and cranial osteopathy offer safe, loving
ways to ease your baby's first months and help
to cope with minor problems that may develop.

a natural affinity with water

While they are growing in the womb, babies are cushioned in fluid, and once they emerge into the world they seem to have a natural affinity with water. Make the most of this – it offers wonderful opportunities for pleasure, physical and mental development, and enhancing your relationship with your child.

A CAUTIONARY NOTE

Remember always to take extreme care in the presence of water. A baby should never be left alone with water – even for a few seconds. Babies and small children can drown in water that is no more than a few centimetres deep; this includes water in sinks, buckets, lavatory pans, fishponds, ditches and puddles.

WATER BIRTH

Babies' affinity with water begins in the womb, where they are constantly bathed in protective amniotic fluid, and continues when they emerge into the world.

Many women who are about to give birth have an instinctive feeling that immersing themselves in water can ease the process of labour. Water births have potential advantages for babies too, including shorter labour, fewer drugs and other interventions, and reduced birth trauma. Mothers who give birth in water tend to be more relaxed than those who do not, so fewer stress hormones are transmitted to the baby.

A water birth tends to generate an atmosphere that is calm and supportive. It also provides the father with an opportunity to play an active role – and the whole experience can enhance family ties.

BATHING

Even the tiniest babies usually enjoy being in water. A bath can be soothing or exciting, depending on the time of day. Water cushions the baby's weight and offers different sensations and experiences – as well as all the fun of water play that can help to develop hand-eye coordination and motor skills.

Remember that newborns need you to support their head at all times – and always test the temperature of the bath water before putting your baby in, to make sure that it is not too hot.

Many babies like to be massaged at bathtime, and adding a few drops of essential oils to a bath is one of the most effective ways to deliver aromatherapy for babies. An aromatherapy bath may be a helpful pre-bedtime ritual, especially since a baby is often relaxed and sleepy after a bath, but massage is a stimulant, so avoid massaging your baby for at least half an hour before bedtime. For more information on baby massage, see pages 24–51; for information on baby aromatherapy, see pages 86–99.

Games at bathtime are an excellent way for fathers to establish a close relationship with their babies and to experience early play. Try gentle splashing games, and

warm water offers a **secure and gentle** environment that may remind babies of what it felt like **in the womb**

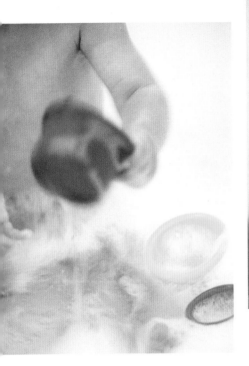

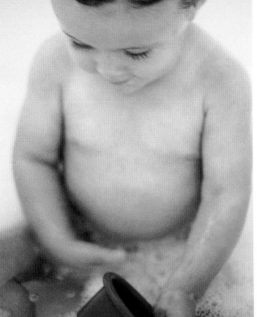

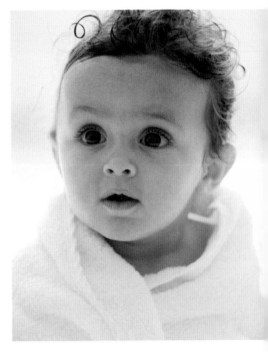

'Caro was never happier than when under water. I think it gave her a great sense of freedom and control.'

PENELOPE, MOTHER OF CARO

let your baby enjoy the textures of bubbles, soap and sponges. Older babies love water toys. You don't need to buy expensive gadgets – as well as small plastic toys such as ducks or boats, experiment with plastic cups and beakers for filling and pouring, and see what fun you can create with sieves, funnels or squeezy bottles.

SWIMMING

If your baby loves being in water, you may want to sign up for a baby swimming course at your local pool or leisure centre. Although babies will not be able to swim on the surface yet – the strength and skills needed for that do not develop until around the age of three – they are capable of swimming short distances under water. This is because babies have a reflex that prompts them to hold their breath under water. This experience

can be very empowering for babies, offering a degree of movement and control over their bodies that is not yet possible on land.

Swimming classes are especially helpful for children with developmental problems such as Down's syndrome or cerebral palsy. They are also marvellous exercise and can do much to help your baby develop self-confidence and coordination, as well as confidence in the water that will pay dividends in years to come.

Classes are available for babies from just a few days old. You don't need to be able to swim yourself – you can simply support your baby while standing in the water. If your local pool doesn't offer baby swimming classes, you may be able to find a local course via the internet by visiting www.waterbabies.co.uk. Avoid lessons for a few days immediately after a vaccination.

'Cranial osteopathy involves an incredibly light touch. I was told by the woman who saw Josh that the pressure applied is usually no more than five grams — about the weight of a twenty-pence piece.'

FENELLA, MOTHER OF LUCINDA AND JOSH

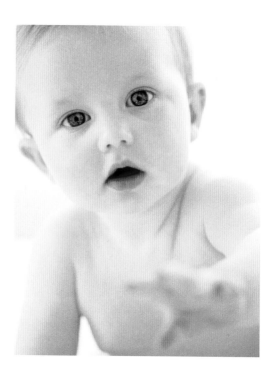

cranial osteopathy

Cranial osteopathy involves gentle manipulation of the bones of the skull to release tensions and relieve various ailments. It may be especially useful in babies to help correct any lingering problems associated with the birth.

OTHER GENTLE THERAPIES

WHEN IS IT NECESSARY?

Cranial osteopathy is a specialized form of osteopathy, a system of manipulation of the skeleton that is designed to detect and correct minor imbalances and to promote optimal mechanical function. Practitioners of cranial osteopathy apply these principles to the skull or, in craniosacral therapy, to the skull and spine right down to the sacrum or tailbone.

During birth, enormous force is exerted on the baby's head as it is pushed and twisted through the bony canal of the mother's pelvis. The still-developing bones of the skull are moulded during this passage down the birth canal. If birth is too rapid, there may be insufficient time for proper moulding of the head to occur. This can also happen in a caesarean delivery, where the baby is suddenly removed from the womb.

On the other hand, a prolonged or difficult labour increases the stress on the baby and the pressures on the head, especially with a forceps or ventouse delivery. These instruments can squash, stretch or bruise the head, creating even greater distortions.

Such forces may make it harder for the baby's bones to settle naturally after birth, and more difficult for the body to self-correct any minor deficiencies. Any remaining tension or grating puts stress on the nervous system, leading potentially to long-term problems.

104

Cranial osteopathy can be beneficial at any age. However, the after-effects of birth trauma are most easily corrected during infancy, before the plates of bone that make up the skull fuse together.

WHAT ARE THE BENEFITS?

Practitioners say that, by correcting subtle imbalances, cranial osteopathy is especially useful in overcoming the effects of difficult births, especially in babies who display behaviours such as persistent crying, irritability or restlessness, and sleeping or feeding difficulties. It can also help to avert later tendencies to asthma or persistent ear or sinus infections. It may also alleviate some of the problems associated with conditions such as Down's syndrome and cerebral palsy.

Cranial osteopathy can also have a beneficial effect on many common conditions of early life, from colic or respiratory problems to learning and behavioural difficulties. For example:

□ An irritable baby who cries or screams a lot may be uncomfortable as the result of a feeling of constant pressure in the head because of distortions of the skull following birth.

□ Feeding difficulties may be caused by mechanical stresses around the face and throat, or nerve irritation affecting the tongue and throat and interfering with the sucking mechanism.

□ A baby who sleeps poorly and wakes up easily may be suffering from tension inside the skull, putting the nervous system in a state of continual alertness.

□ Infant colic, excessive wind or milk regurgitation may be due to irritation of the nerves passing to the stomach and diaphragm, resulting in poor digestion.

WHAT HAPPENS DURING A CONSULTATION?

Cranial osteopaths begin by feeling the skull for any restrictions, patterns of tension or pressure build-up. They then use a combination of massage and very gentle manipulation to correct any imbalances. Patients stay fully clothed during the session, although they take off their shoes.

Babies usually respond well to cranial osteopathy, and because the treatment is so gentle, it is virtually free of side effects.

Some babies may become more restless for a time, which usually passes after a day or so. More often, they become rapidly calmer after a treatment and may sleep more soundly almost at once. A series of treatments may be needed to correct deeper imbalances.

CHOOSING A PRACTITIONER

If you think that your baby might benefit from cranial osteopathy, you will need to consult a professional therapist. The Sutherland Society is the UK's largest organization devoted to cranial osteopathy, and all their members have completed recognized postgraduate training. Find local members of the Sutherland Society on its website: www.cranial.org.uk. Alternatively, contact the Sutherland Cranial College or the General Osteopathic Council (see page 124).

many **after-effects of birth** are hard to distinguish from normal baby behaviour; only by trying **cranial osteopathy** can you know whether **it helps** your baby

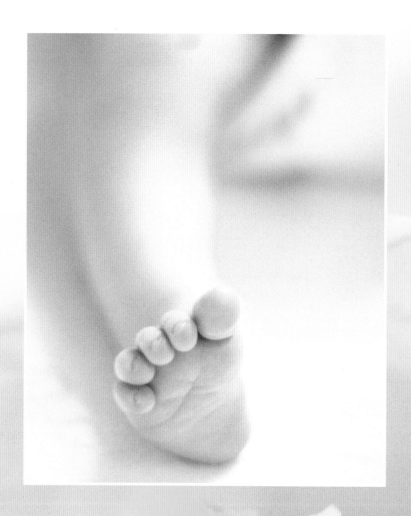

pressure on the different **'reflex areas'** of the foot
stimulates **nerve endings** and promotes
relaxation . . . it is a wonderful way to show **your love**

reflexology for babies

Like most parents, you have probably marvelled on occasion at your baby's tiny feet. If you use reflexology regularly, those perfect little appendages could hold the key to calmer days and more restful nights.

HOW REFLEXOLOGY WORKS

Reflexology is a system of foot massage based on the belief that parts of the body are mirrored in the sole of the foot. Pressure on the different 'reflex areas' on the foot stimulates nerve endings and promotes relaxation.

Although it does not treat diseases, reflexology is thought to improve energy flow, balance function and enhance healing in the corresponding part of the body. Foot massage also boosts circulation and toxin release, improves digestion and excretion and promotes vitality.

Babies and children respond very well – and rapidly – to reflexology. Like body massage, it is a wonderful way to communicate and show your love for your baby, as well as being soothing – and fun to do! As your child grows older, you may be able to use reflexology to relieve any build-up of stress and tension, though some toddlers simply find it impossible to sit still for long enough. Others may want to massage you in return!

HOW DO I USE REFLEXOLOGY ON A BABY?

The answer is: very, very gently. Reflexology in adults and children over the age of five requires reasonably firm pressure, but when you massage a baby's or toddler's feet you need a feather-like touch. As long as the baby is enjoying it, you can do no harm.

Some babies find the sensation of having their feet massaged strange – if they withdraw their feet or seem uncomfortable, stop and try again on another occasion.

You may find that your baby has a bowel movement immediately after a reflexology session – this shows that it has worked to promote elimination.

GUIDELINES

Here are some guidelines for baby reflexology:
□ Make the atmosphere warm and cosy.
□ Play some calming background music, if you like.
□ Imagine the foot divided into five zones running up and down the sole. Start with the outer band and stroke from heel to toe, then move on to the next and work each one in turn.
□ Use a stroking touch with your thumb, or use only a fingertip until your baby is a few weeks old.
□ Give light strokes, always moving up the foot and working gradually from heel to toe.
□ Short and frequent is the best approach – you can massage the whole foot in a couple of minutes.
□ Work each foot in turn.

WHAT CONDITIONS CAN REFLEXOLOGY HELP?

Parents report that, in addition to its calming effect, reflexology helps babies to recover from a difficult birth. Some have also found that it can alleviate any tendency to hyperactivity. In addition, using reflexology on specific areas of the feet is claimed to help the body to deal with various minor ailments, as described in the Healthy and Calm chapter (pages 114–23).

If your baby has a tendency to any common ailments, you may wish to consider consulting a professional reflexologist, although a few gentle reflexology sessions at home will do no harm if you wish to try these first.

Remember that you should always seek medical advice for all but the most trivial ailment – or if simple home treatments don't help within a few days.

homeopathy for babies

Based on the principle of 'like cures like', homeopathic remedies are extremely dilute preparations of substances that would cause similar symptoms if administered in full dose.

SAFE HEALING

Homeopathy offers safe, gentle healing for minor baby ailments. The remedies are so dilute that they have no side effects and pose no danger. They do not interact with orthodox medicines, so you can use homeopathy alongside conventional treatment, but tell your doctor in advance. Unlike conventional drugs, homeopathic remedies are chosen to match not only the symptoms but also the physical and emotional characteristics of the sufferer. However, some remedies are commonly used for certain situations, and many are available from high-street pharmacies and health-food shops, although you may choose to see a practitioner to gain the most benefit, or if home treatment is not helping.

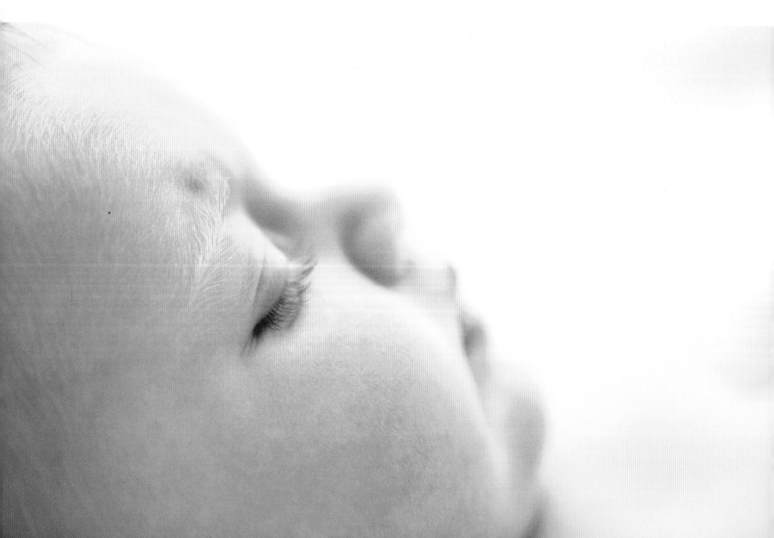

WHAT CONDITIONS CAN HOMEOPATHY HELP?

Many women use homeopathic remedies in pregnancy to ensure optimal health before the birth and to treat symptoms such as heartburn without exposing their foetus to the side effects of medical drugs.

After birth, babies too must cope with major bodily changes as well as a range of new sensations and experiences. Homeopathic remedies can reduce shock or stress, help to calm a fretful baby and alleviate the effects of allergies. They are used to treat earache, eczema and minor ailments such as coughs and colds, as well as sleeping, feeding and digestive problems.

Some specific remedies are suggested in the Healthy and Calm chapter (pages 114–23).

USING HOMEOPATHIC REMEDIES

Most homeopathic remedies come as tiny tablets called pillules. The strength of a remedy is believed to increase each time it is diluted – so the 30C potency, which has been diluted more, is stronger than 6C. (C stands for Centesimal, meaning a one-hundred-fold dilution.)
□ Start with 6C potency.
□ If using tablets, crush them in a clean teaspoon and place the powder under the baby's tongue to dissolve.
□ If you are breastfeeding, you can take the remedy yourself (at 6C potency) rather than give it to the baby.
□ Give one dose three times daily for up to three days. Stop when symptoms improve.
□ Avoid feeding for 30 minutes before or after a dose.
□ Store remedies in a cool, dark place.

HOW DO I KNOW WHEN TO SEEK FURTHER HELP?

Always seek medical advice for any but the most minor health problem in a baby, especially if it involves a change in behaviour or alertness, or difficulty with feeding or breathing.

After using a homeopathic remedy, it is common for symptoms to get worse before they get better – this

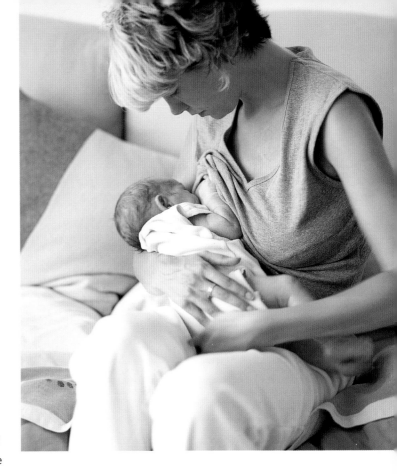

shows that the body is responding to the remedy and preparing to heal. But, if minor symptoms increase to a worrying level, or if there is no improvement after three days, stop using the remedy and seek help.

BENEFITS IN THE EARLY DAYS

In the early days and weeks after birth, your baby may benefit from the following remedies.
□ To help recovery from the intense experience of birth: Aconite.
□ For bruising resulting from a prolonged or difficult birth, especially a forceps delivery: Arnica.
□ For healing an inflamed belly button: Silica.
□ For soothing an irritable baby who dislikes being picked up: Bryonia.
□ For calming a tearful, snuffly baby who is not sleeping well at night: Merc. sol.
□ For a tired and emotional baby who regularly produces a lot of mucus: Pulsatilla.

bach flower remedies

The 38 Bach Flower Remedies are named after Dr Edward Bach, a medical doctor and homeopath practising in the early 20th century, who believed that emotional imbalance is the cause of many physical ailments, and that the healing vibrations of certain flowers and other plants can restore energy balance and harmony.

WHAT ARE BACH FLOWER REMEDIES?

The remedies are liquid essences derived from plants. They are prepared by floating or boiling the plant parts in spring water, then preserving in 50–50 mix with alcohol (usually brandy). These 'mother tinctures' are further diluted with alcohol before bottling. They are sold in health-food shops and are intended to be simple enough to use at home, but you may wish to consult a practitioner for complex problems. The remedies are not meant to treat serious medical problems. If simple home treatments are not working, or you are at all worried about your baby, seek medical advice promptly.

HOW TO USE THE REMEDIES

□ Dilute according to instructions – generally 2 to 3 drops in 20 to 30ml water.

□ Use up to six remedies at once, if necessary – add them all to the same water.

□ Place diluted remedies directly on the tongue or on lips, temples, wrists or behind the ears. Once the baby is weaned, you can add flower remedies to food or drinks.

□ Use up to 4 drops of diluted remedy four times a day. You may need to continue for four days for a short-term problem or ten days for a temperamental issue.

□ Stock remedies keep for months in a cool, dark place. Diluted solutions should be kept for two weeks at most.

RESCUE REMEDY

Perhaps the best known preparation of this type is Rescue Remedy, which is in fact a combination of five Flower Remedies: Cherry Plum (for inability to cope), Clematis (for inattentiveness), Impatiens (for irritation and impatience), Rock Rose (for terror) and Star of Bethlehem (for the after-effects of shock).

Rescue Remedy is recommended by practitioners for use in any traumatic situation, whether physical or psychological, including the after-effects of birth trauma (for the mother as well as the baby). You may find it effective in calming an older child following a tantrum or accident. Rescue Remedy cream includes the five ingredients listed above plus Crab Apple (for physical and psychological cleansing).

In an emergency, Rescue Remedy can be taken straight from the stock bottle. Otherwise, give 4 drops in water, to sip at intervals, or place on the skin.

WHAT CONDITIONS CAN THE REMEDIES HELP?

Each of the 38 Flower Remedies deals with a particular mental state. Some that are especially helpful in babies are listed below. Other specific remedies for common childhood ailments are suggested in the Healthy and Calm chapter (see pages 114–23).

□ For fearful or timid babies: Mimulus.

□ For impatient or irritable babies: Impatiens, Rescue Remedy.

□ For babies who need continual attention: Chicory.

□ For babies who are always active and find it hard to settle: Vervain.

□ For frustrated babies who seem to scream with fury: Cherry Plum, Rescue Remedy.

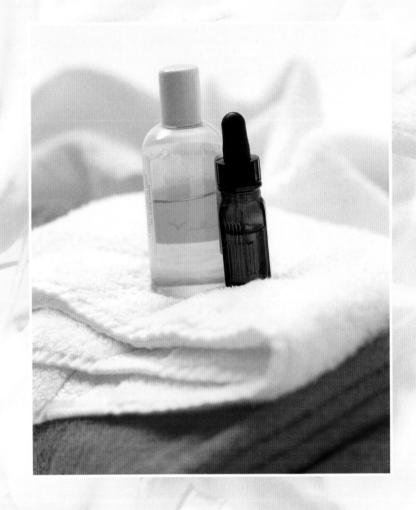

as in homeopathy, **flower remedies** are chosen on the
basis of an individual's personality and **emotional
state** as much as to treat **specific symptoms**

New parents face a profusion of advice about sleep. What sort of night-time routine is best? Should your baby sleep in your bed, in a cot in your room, or in another room alone? Should you leave a baby to cry or not? Whatever you decide, bear in mind that, generally, babies take as much sleep as they need – lack of sleep is largely a problem for parents, not for the baby!

TEN WAYS TO... *get a good night's sleep*

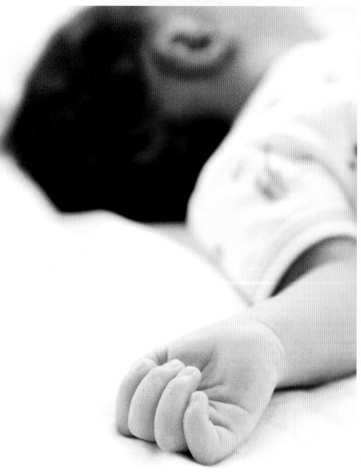

1 Babies need to learn the difference between night and day. If necessary, heighten the distinction between the two by hanging thick curtains or blackout blinds at bedroom windows.

2 After about six weeks of age, start to establish a regular bedtime routine – for example, bath your baby, dress in nightclothes, give a feed, tell a story or sing a lullaby, and kiss goodnight. Keep to the same routine each night.

3 Make sleeping spaces slightly cooler than daytime rooms: 18° to 21°C (65° to 70°F) is ideal.

4 Use aromatherapy to get your baby into a sleepy mood. The essential oils for inducing sleepiness are chamomile and lavender. Either diffuse 1 drop of chamomile and 2 drops of lavender in the baby's room (see page 90) or add 1 drop of chamomile and 1 drop of lavender to one teaspoon of full-fat milk and mix into a warm bath (see page 92).

5 Have a 'winding-down' period and avoid over-stimulating your baby for at least an hour before bedtime. Install a dimmer switch in the baby's room so you can lower the lighting levels whenever you need to.

6 Babies become accustomed to a certain level of background noise in the womb, which is why many sleep well while the vacuum cleaner or dishwasher is running. Consider playing a CD of white noise, nature sounds or some soothing classical music to help your baby to drift off.

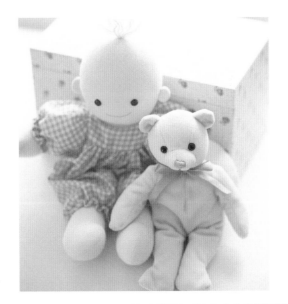

7 Babies who wake in the night should have their needs attended to, but try to avoid waking them even more: talk in whispers, avoid eye contact, keep lighting level to the minimum you need to see what you are doing, gently change or feed, then put back to sleep.

8 While your baby still sleeps during the day, watch for individual signs that mean 'I'm tired' – such as rubbing the eyes, pulling on the ears or drooping of the eyelids – and settle him or her down for a nap at once. If you leave it too long, the baby may become overtired and find it difficult to get to sleep.

9 Move your baby into strong natural daylight as soon as possible in the morning – preferably outside in the sunshine or near a window – and take outdoors into the fresh air for at least two hours each day.

10 Regular massage improves babies' sleeping patterns and helps them to fall asleep more quickly, but massage stimulates the nervous system so a baby will not necessarily fall asleep straight after a massage. It is the frequency of massage, rather than the timing, that helps with sleep, so massage babies when they are wide awake, not when they are tired.

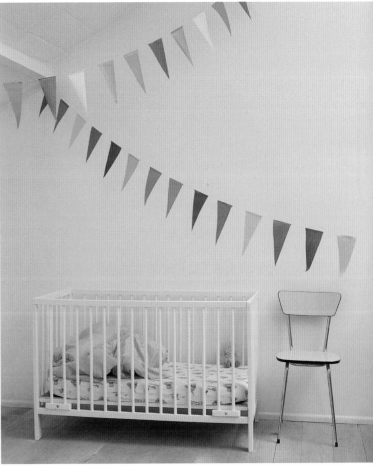

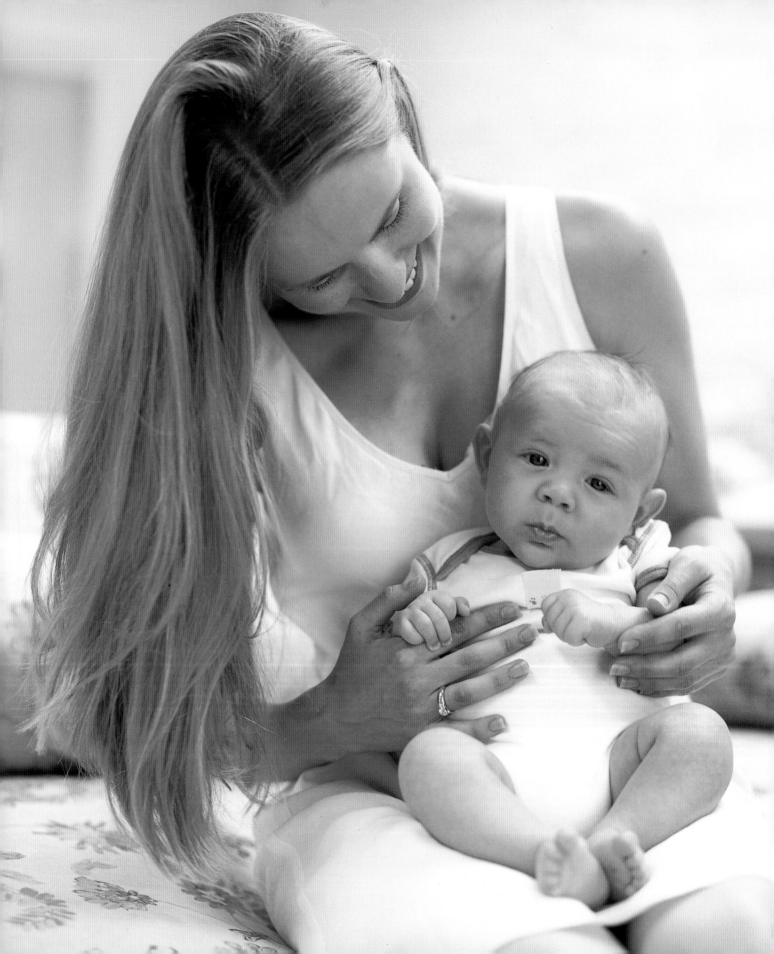

healthy and calm

All babies will succumb to various minor ailments. Most – such as snuffles, coughs and colds – are self-limiting, and your baby simply needs plenty of loving attention and perhaps some of the gentle remedies suggested in this chapter. Always be alert, though, for those times when you should seek medical attention. If in doubt, ask for help.

your baby's health

There are few things more worrying or upsetting for a parent than the illness of a baby or child. Your first thought is always likely to be: 'Is it serious?' The answer is often hard to discover, especially in the case of children who are too young to tell you how they are feeling.

WHEN TO SEEK MEDICAL ADVICE

Parents need to be vigilant about illness in babies and toddlers, since their bodily systems are still immature, with the result that complications may prove more threatening than they would be in older children or adults. If a child's temperature rises above 40°C (104°F), call a doctor at once. As a general rule, seek urgent attention for any illness where your baby or toddler is:

□ Floppy, lethargic or difficult to rouse.

□ Seems in severe pain.

□ Has an unusually high-pitched or strange cry.

□ Has trouble breathing.

□ Has a high temperature.

□ Has fits or seizures.

□ Cannot feed properly for more than a day.

□ Has profuse diarrhoea or vomiting.

□ Shows signs of dehydration – sunken eyes, loose dry skin and floppy limbs.

□ Has a sudden or unexplained worsening of symptoms.

□ Loses weight.

□ Bleeds from any orifice.

Ultimately, the most constructive advice may be to trust your instincts. If you believe that something is not right with your baby, seek professional help promptly.

BE PREPARED

Since there are many things that will inevitably worry you as a parent, it makes sense to be well prepared to deal with a variety of health problems. Start by finding a doctor and other healthcare professionals whom you trust. Invest in a good first-aid book and a good home medical guide, ideally one that covers both conventional and complementary medicines, if this fits your preferred approach. Ensure that you have supplies of remedies you would choose for common conditions such as colds or nappy rash.

LOVE AND SECURITY

For the many minor ailments that are an inevitable part of growing up, you as a parent can actually supply the best medicine there is – love combined with warmth, security and nourishing food. Whenever a child is feeling ill or out of sorts, touch is vital. Don't forget the

it is part of the **challenge** of nurturing to supply the most effective **mixture of ingredients** for a child's healthy development: **love, warmth** and **security**

'When Guy was a baby, I used to get frantic with worry every time he had a cold or seemed a bit off-colour. By the time Angie was born, I had come to realize that minor ailments are just a part of growing up.'

CAMILLE, MOTHER OF GUY, FREDDIE AND ANGIE

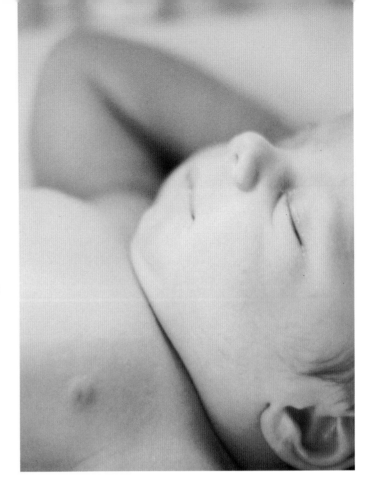

therapeutic power of a loving hug and the fact that cuddles can help, if not heal. If you are breastfeeding, keep it up – as well as giving nourishment, it protects against infections and allergies, and reassures your baby by providing physical contact and an affirmation of your love. Once a baby is weaned, offer plenty to drink and whatever soothing, nutritious foods your baby likes.

HOME TREATMENTS
There are many remedies suggested in this book that can be used safely on babies. When dealing with short-term trauma or illness, Rescue Remedy (see page 110) may help almost anything. Massage and reflexology are generally soothing and can help to take the edge off symptoms and make a fractious baby feel more relaxed and secure. For longer-term problems, it may be worth asking a cranial osteopath to examine your baby, to see if there are any after-effects of birth trauma and if

anything can be done to alleviate them (see pages 104–105). You may also like to consider consulting a homeopath (see pages 108–109).

Remember, though, that many symptoms have a purpose. Some are a form of communication – nappy rash tells you that your baby's skin needs more fresh air; diarrhoea may suggest that a breastfeeding mother needs to avoid a particular food; and sleeping problems may hint that your baby is not getting enough light and fresh air during the day. Often, symptoms represent the body's own healing process, which is more potent than any medicine. For example, a fever may be the body's clever response to invading bacteria or viruses, which are killed off at higher temperatures.

Your baby's own body will do most of the work of getting better. Gentle remedies – along with loving touch and healthy nourishment – may help to support or stimulate these natural healing powers.

'Mathew seemed to be in genuine pain when his bottom side teeth started coming through. I found that gently massaging his jawline with my fingertips really helped to soothe him.'

NATASHA, MOTHER OF JOHN AND MATHEW

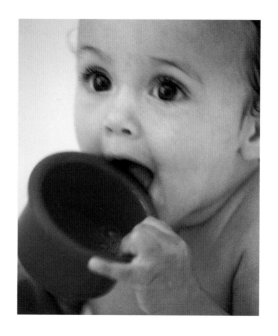

relieving minor ailments

Here are some suggestions for dealing with the most common ailments your child is likely to encounter in the early years. For more information on cranial osteopathy, reflexology, homeopathic remedies and Bach Flower Remedies, see pages 104–111.

BUMPS AND BRUISES

Once your baby begins to crawl and, later, to walk, bumps and bruises are inevitable.

□ Hold an ice pack wrapped in a towel against the bruised skin for ten minutes.

□ Try homeopathic remedies: Arnica or Calendula cream.

□ Try Rescue Remedy cream.

BURNS

Babies' delicate skin burns relatively easily, and even sunburn can have serious consequences. A common cause of burns in babies is scalding from hot liquids. Never carry a baby at the same time as a hot drink.

□ Immediate first aid: flush the area with cold water for at least ten minutes. Seek medical help for any burn that looks nasty, blisters or covers an area bigger than the baby's hand. Call an ambulance for serious burns.

□ Never put anything greasy or oily on a burn for the first 48 hours; it simply seals in the heat.

□ Soothing remedies include cool (not cold) baths and aloe vera gel, from a cut leaf or a proprietary product.

□ For a small burn, apply 1 drop of neat lavender essential oil to the affected area. (Normally, essential oils should never be used neat on a baby.)

□ Try homeopathic remedies: for shock, Aconite; to promote healing, Arnica; for sunburn, Belladonna.

□ Try Rescue Remedy cream.

COLDS AND COUGHS

An average healthy baby has six colds before the age of one. Encountering new viruses and bacteria develops immunity, but colds can precede more serious problems. If symptoms worsen, the baby's body temperature rises above 38°C (100.4°F) – a normal temperature is about 37°C (98.6°F) – or you are worried, call a doctor.

□ Use a vaporizer in order to humidify the air and loosen sticky mucus.

□ Massage your baby's head and face to clear a blocked nose and to prevent colds (see pages 40–41).

□ Massage your baby's chest to improve lung function (see pages 36–37).

□ Try aromatherapy: diffuse lavender and myrtle essential oils in your baby's room (see page 90).

□ Try homeopathic remedies: for treating a runny nose, Allium cepa or Belladonna; for thick mucus, Pulsatilla; for congestion with difficulty feeding, Nux vomica; for a chesty cough with mucus, Hepar. sulph.

□ Try reflexology: massage your baby just under the fleshy bits of the toe pads (the reflex area for the sinuses), the middle inside edges of the big toes (the nose) and the balls of the feet (the lungs).

□ For treating persistent snuffles in a baby, avoid cow's milk and cow's milk products.

COLIC

Colic – inconsolable crying for hours, usually in the evenings – is miserable for both babies and parents. Consult your doctor to make sure that your baby has no underlying problem.

□ If you are breastfeeding, avoid dairy products and spices and drink chamomile tea.

□ Swaddle your baby (see page 13).

□ Give your baby a warm bath or put a well-wrapped hot-water bottle next to the baby's abdominal area.

□ Carry your baby in the 'kangaroo' position (see page 17) in a quiet, dimly lit environment; colic may be linked with difficulty in making the transition between alertness and sleepiness.

□ Swing your baby in the Tiger in a Tree position to relieve any wind (see pages 60–61).

□ Massage your baby's abdominal area (see pages 36–37) with a mixture of dill and mandarin essential oils diluted in almond or grapeseed oil (see page 95).

□ Try reflexology: massage the outer edges of the soles between the pad of the heel and the middle of the foot (the reflex area for the colon or large intestine).

□ Consider cranial osteopathy; consult a practitioner.

□ Try homeopathic remedies: for fretful crying, Chamomilla; for colic that gets worse after feeding, Nux vomica; for greenish stools and sleeping problems associated with colic, Nat. phos.

□ Try Bach Flower Remedies: Rock Rose or Rescue Remedy cream applied to the abdomen.

□ Give tiny doses of sugar water. Dissolve a teaspoon of sugar in about 100ml boiled water and leave to cool. Drop it slowly into your baby's mouth with a dropper or teaspoon. It soothes colic in some babies and can't harm teeth before they come through.

CONSTIPATION

Constipation is unusual in babies, especially in breastfed infants, although it may affect babies taking bottled milk or solid food for the first time.

See your doctor if your baby doesn't pass faeces for four days – or immediately if there is pain.

□ Increase a weaned baby's fluid intake.

□ Offer fresh pears or stewed prune juice to a weaned baby. If you are breastfeeding, take these yourself.

□ Massage your baby's abdominal area (see pages 36–37) with a mixture of dill and mandarin essential oils diluted in almond or grapeseed oil (see page 95).

□ Try reflexology: massage the outer edges of the soles between the pad of the heel and the middle of the foot (the reflex area for the colon or large intestine).

'I know that some people are sceptical about the effectiveness of homeopathic remedies, but I found they were the only thing that did anything to help my children's eczema.'

NAOMI, MOTHER OF JULIAN AND CHRISTOPHER

□ Swing your baby gently in the Tiger in a Tree position (see pages 60–61).
□ Try homeopathic remedies: to relieve irritation, Nux vomica; after a fever, Bryonia or Sulphur.
□ Try Bach Flower Remedies: Walnut or Holly.

CRADLE CAP

A patch of yellow, waxy, scaly skin on top of your baby's scalp is caused by excess oil production. It usually goes away without treatment. If it bothers you:
□ Avoid bathcare products for babies (see page 21).
□ Spread a little olive oil over the patch, wait ten minutes, then gently brush it off with a baby brush or flannel. For a severe case, leave on overnight.
□ Try aromatherapy: apply benzoin and lavender essential oils diluted in jojoba oil to your baby's scalp (see page 95).
□ Try homeopathic remedies: Sulphur or Rhus. tox.

DIARRHOEA

Diarrhoea is common in babies. If it is prolonged, and especially if it is accompanied by fever with a body temperature above 38°C (100.4°F), your baby risks becoming dehydrated. Call a doctor if diarrhoea in a baby lasts more than two days.

□ If you are breastfeeding, avoid drinking fruit juices.
□ Try reflexology: massage the outer edges of the soles between the pad of the heel and the middle of the foot (the reflex area for the colon or large intestine).
□ Try homeopathic remedies: for adverse food reactions or offensive stools, Arsen. alb.; if fever accompanies diarrhoea, Belladonna; if the baby has a good appetite despite persistent diarrhoea, Sulphur; if diarrhoea coincides with teething, Chamomilla.
□ Try a Bach Flower Remedy: Walnut.

EARACHE

Earache may follow a cold. Your baby will seem irritable and distracted, often tugging at one ear. If your baby seems in severe pain or develops a fever with a body temperature above 38°C (100.4°F), seek medical help.
□ Try reflexology: massage the underside of the middle toes at the point where the toes join the ball of the foot (the reflex area for the ear points).
□ To combat chronic infection (known as 'glue ear'), consider cranial osteopathy plus homeopathy; for each therapy, consult a practitioner.
□ Sometimes babies put foreign objects such as raisins into their ears. Do not try to remove such an object; instead, seek medical help.

ECZEMA AND DRY SKIN

Skin reactions are common in babies because of their delicate skin. If a reaction persists, blisters or becomes infected, consult a doctor.

□ Avoid perfumed or medicated bath products.

□ Use a simple emollient such as aqueous cream for baths and moisturizing.

□ Put plain cotton mittens on your baby's hands to discourage scratching.

□ Try homeopathic remedies: for dry, flaky, itchy skin, Arsen. alb.; for cracked, weeping skin, Graphites.

□ Try Bach Flower Remedies: for fretfulness with itching, Impatiens or Rock Rose.

If there is a family history of eczema:

□ Avoid giving cow's milk, eggs, wheat-based products or nuts until your baby is at least a year old.

□ In your baby's bedroom, have a solid floor covering rather than carpets, and blinds instead of curtains.

□ Wash bedding regularly on a hot setting and put soft toys in the freezer overnight to kill dust mites.

□ Don't keep pets.

FEEDING AND DIGESTIVE PROBLEMS

Any illness can put a baby off feeding. Call a doctor if your baby cannot feed properly for more than a day.

□ For breastfeeding problems, seek help from the La Leche League or the National Childbirth Trust.

□ Consider cranial osteopathy; consult a practitioner.

□ Try reflexology: massage the hollow of the foot in the middle of the sole, especially the inner edges (the reflex areas for the liver, stomach and intestinal area).

□ Try a homeopathic remedy: if feeding problems are due to thrush, Borax (for both of you).

FEVERS

Always seek medical attention for a small baby whose body temperature rises above 38°C (100.4°F), the most obvious symptom of a fever.

□ For a high fever, sponge the baby with tepid water until the doctor arrives.

□ Try homeopathic remedies: for a fever with restlessness, Aconite; for a fever with crying, Pulsatilla; for a fever in reaction to an immunization, Silica; for persistent fever, Kali. phos.

□ Try Bach Flower Remedies: Impatiens or Rock Rose.

NAPPY RASH

The most effective cure for nappy rash is to do without nappies! Whenever possible, allow your baby to play naked – in the garden in summer, or on a solid floor or leakproof mat in winter.

□ Try aromatherapy: apply 1 drop of chamomile or 1 drop of lavender essential oil diluted in one dessertspoon of jojoba oil to the affected area (see page 95).

□ Try a homeopathic remedy: Calendula cream.

□ Try Bach Flower Remedies: Sulphur or Rescue Remedy cream.

SLEEPING PROBLEMS

Some babies are naturally inclined to sleep more deeply and for longer periods than others, and all babies are more likely to sleep poorly at certain times – for

colic may be linked with difficulty in **making the transition** between alertness and **sleepiness**

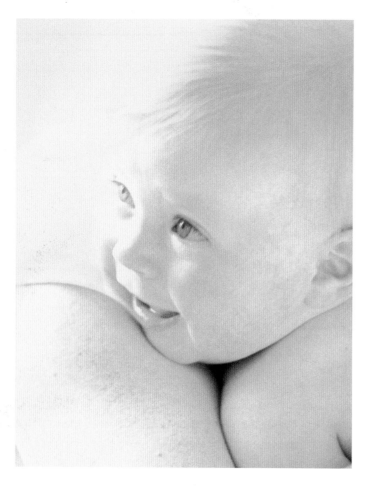

example, when they are teething or suffering from an illness, or after immunizations. See pages 112–13 for suggestions on how to promote sound sleep.

☐ If you are breastfeeding, avoid caffeine and other stimulants.

☐ Massage your baby's face (see pages 40–41).

☐ Try aromatherapy: diffuse chamomile and lavender essential oils in your baby's room (see page 90) or add them to bedtime bathwater (see page 92).

☐ Consider cranial osteopathy for long-term sleeping problems; consult a practitioner.

☐ Try homeopathic remedies: for waking with symptoms that resemble colic, Carbo. veg. or China; for difficulty falling asleep followed by waking alert, Chamomilla; for short-term night-waking after a fright or trauma, Arnica.

☐ Try Bach Flower Remedies: for fretfulness, Rock Rose or Impatiens; for babies who don't sleep much, White Chestnut or Rescue Remedy; for fear of the dark, Aspen.

STICKY EYE

Minor eye infections, caused by tiny and immature tear ducts, are common in babies.

☐ Washing regularly with tepid water should help to prevent infections.

☐ Mother's milk is one of the best cures. It contains lysosomes, the infection-fighting substances in tears, and is safe to use as an eyewash.

☐ Try reflexology: massage the underside of your baby's second toes (the reflex area for the eyes).

☐ Try a homeopathic remedy: especially for irritable babies prone to colds, Silica.

TEETHING PROBLEMS

You can often tell a tooth is coming if the child is irritable and dribbling, with a red, flushed face.

☐ Massage your baby's face (see pages 40–41).

☐ Massage your baby's gums with your finger after first dipping the finger in lemon juice (see page 51).

☐ Try reflexology: massage the inside edges of the base of your baby's big toes (the reflex area for the mouth).

☐ Try Bach Flower Remedies: Walnut or Red Chestnut.

☐ Try Chamomilla teething granules or over-the-counter teething gel.

☐ Try cool teething rings or cold foods and drinks.

☐ Apply barrier cream to the chin to prevent soreness from dribbling.

WIND

Trapped wind, which can cause a lot of discomfort, may be effectively relieved by gentle movement.

☐ Massage your baby's abdomen (see pages 36–37).

☐ Try swinging your baby in the Tiger in a Tree position (see pages 60–61).

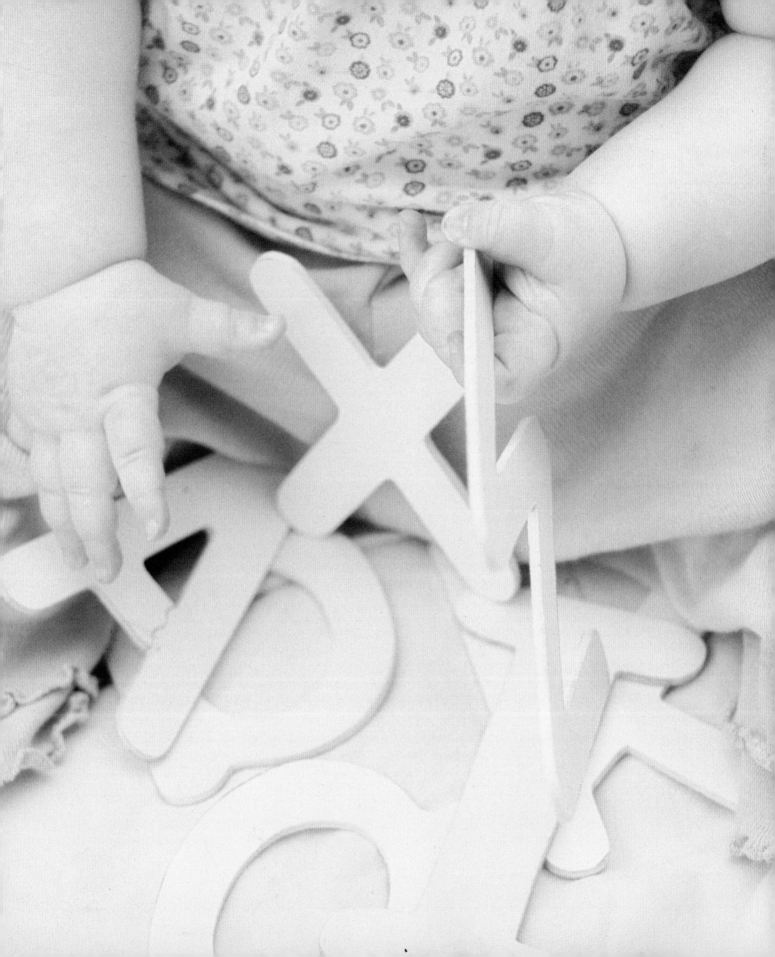

useful addresses

Baby Directory
020 8678 9000
www.babydirectory.com
*Regional directories of
baby-related activities,
including massage classes.*

**British Reflexology
Association**
Monks Orchard
Whitbourne
Worcestershire WR6 5RB
01886 821207
www.britreflex.co.uk
*Visit the website to find
a reflexologist near you.*

Daycare Trust
21 St George's Road
London SE1 6ES
childcare hotline:
020 7840 3350
www.daycaretrust.org.uk
*Charity that promotes high-
quality childcare for all.*

Dr Edward Bach Centre
Mount Vernon
Bakers Lane
Sotwell
Oxfordshire OX10 0PZ
01491 834678
www.bachcentre.com
*Information about Bach
Flower Remedies and
how to obtain them.*

Enata
PO Box 830A
Thames Ditton
Surrey KT1 9BB
www.enata.co.uk
020 8339 0696
Aromatherapy supplies.

**General
Osteopathic Council**
Osteopathy House
176 Tower Bridge Road
London SE1 3LU
020 7357 6655
www.osteopathy.org.uk
*Visit the website to find
an osteopath near you.*

**International Federation
of Aromatherapists (IFA)**
61–63 Churchfield Road
London W3 6AY
020 8992 8945
*Advice on finding qualified
aromatherapy practitioners
and suppliers.*

**International Therapy
Examination Council (ITEC)**
2nd Floor, Chiswick Gate
508–608 Chiswick High Road
London W4 5RP
020 8994 4141
*Advice on finding qualified
aromatherapy practitioners
and suppliers.*

**La Leche League of
Great Britain**
24-hour helpline:
0845 120 2918
www.laleche.org.uk
*Immediate breastfeeding
support and information.*

Little Me Baby Organics
c/o Florama
Teddington
Middlesex TW11 8EE
www.littleme
babyorganics.co.uk
Baby aromatherapy products.

**National Childbirth Trust
(NCT)**
Alexandra House
Oldham Terrace
London W3 6NH
020 8992 8637
breastfeeding line:
0870 444 8708
www.nctpregnancyand
babycare.com
*Support and advice on all
aspects of birth and babycare,
including local NCT groups.*

**Osteopathic Centre for
Children (OCC)**
www.occ.uk.com
OCC London
The School House
Woodbridge Street
London EC1R 0ND
020 7490 5510
OCC Manchester
Phoenix Mill
Piercy Street, Ancoats
Manchester M4 7HY
0161 277 9911
*Osteopathic treatment for a
wide range of conditions for
children up to the age of 18.*

Parent Network
Room 2
Winchester House
Kennington Park
11 Cranmer Road
London SW9 6EJ
parent enquiry line:
020 7735 1214
*A charity offering parenting
courses run by specially
trained parents.*

Parentline Plus
free national helpline for
parents: 0808 800 2222

Relate
Herbert Grey College
Little Church Street
Rugby
Warwickshire CV21 3AP
helpline: 0870 601 2121
01788 573241
www.relate.org.uk
*Advice on adapting to
life with a new baby.*

**Royal London
Homeopathic Hospital**
60 Great Ormond Street
London WC1N 3HR
020 7837 8833
Includes a children's clinic.

Serene (formerly CRY-SIS)
BM Serene Crysis
London WC1N 3XX
helpline: 020 7404 5011
www.our-space.co.uk/
serene.asp
*Support for families with
excessively crying, sleepless
and demanding babies.*

Society of Homeopaths
11 Brookfield
Duncan Close
Moulton Park
Northampton NN3 6WL
www.homeopathy-soh.com
0845 450 6611
*Visit the website to find
a homeopath near you.*

Sutherland Cranial College
PO Box 91
Chepstow
Gwent NP16 7ZS
01291 689908
www.scc-osteopathy.co.uk
*Visit the website to find a
cranial osteopath near you.*

index

authors' acknowledgments

SHEENA MEREDITH I wish to send love and thanks to my beautiful daughter, Bryony, for enabling me to share her happy babyhood, and for so many joyful times since.

TINA LAM I would like to thank my teacher, Peter Walker, pioneer of baby massage and baby yoga and gym in London.

CLARE MUNDY I am deeply grateful to Carol Hatton and Trudy Kerr and their model babies, Evie and Louis, and to Trudy's daughter, Ruby. A big thank you to all my students, especially Cynthia, Marie, Ana and Tracey, and their babies, Benjamin, Erin, Paolo and twins Hope and Miles; to Kim Robson, my website designer, and to Chris Mullett of www.silenciomusic.co.uk and Trudy Kerr of www.trudykerr.com for supplying sounds. And, lastly, my thanks to Henrietta, Sonya, Dan and Paul for making my participation in this book so enjoyable.

GLENDA TAYLOR Thank you to Ryland Peters & Small for giving me the opportunity again to 'spread the word' regarding aromatherapy. Also thank you to my children for being such shining examples of how aromatherapy can be used naturally and instinctively throughout life.

publishers' acknowledgments

The publishers would like to say thank you to all our lovely models, especially Nasima and Kamran; Kiri, Cleo and Mazi; Rebecca and Ruben; Anna and Loxie; Charlie, Alex and Lula; Vicki and Kiki; Jenn and Leo; Sara, Alfie and Florence; and Joshua. Special thanks as well to Carol and Evie, and to Trudy, Louis and Ruby.

photography credits

Photography by Dan Duchars unless otherwise stated.
key: **a**=above, **b**=below, **r**=right, **l**=left, **ph**=photographer.

Back jacket Debi Treloar; Page **1** © Stockbyte; **2–4** ph Debi Treloar; **5 background** and **b inset** ph Debi Treloar; **13** ph Debi Treloar/ Victoria Andreae's house in London; **15** ph Debi Treloar; **19** © Stockbyte; **20** ph Debi Treloar; **21a** ph Caroline Arber/Emma Bowman Interior Design; **21b** ph Polly Wreford; **44b** © Stockbyte; **45** background and **84** ph David Montgomery; **87** ph Daniel Farmer; **88–89** ph David Montgomery; **92–93** ph Debi Treloar; **94–97** ph David Montgomery; **103** ph Debi Treloar; **104** © Stockbyte; **106** background ph David Montgomery; **106 inset** ph Debi Treloar; **108** © Stockbyte; **111** background ph Christopher Drake; **111 inset** ph David Montgomery; **112 inset** © Stockbyte; **112 background** ph David Montgomery; **113a & b** ph Debi Treloar/ Vincent and Frieda Plasschaerts' house in Bruges, Belgium; **116** ph David Montgomery; **117–28** ph Debi Treloar.